SpringerBriefs in Public Health

SpringerBriefs in Public Health present concise summaries of cutting-edge research and practical applications from across the entire field of public health, with contributions from medicine, bioethics, health economics, public policy, biostatistics, and sociology.

The focus of the series is to highlight current topics in public health of interest to a global audience, including health care policy; social determinants of health; health issues in developing countries; new research methods; chronic and infectious disease epidemics; and innovative health interventions.

Featuring compact volumes of 55 to 125 pages, the series covers a range of content from professional to academic. Possible volumes in the series may consist of timely reports of state-of-the art analytical techniques, reports from the field, snapshots of hot and/or emerging topics, literature reviews, and in-depth case studies. Both solicited and unsolicited manuscripts are considered for publication in this series.

Briefs are published as part of Springer's eBook collection, with millions of users worldwide. In addition, Briefs are available for individual print and electronic purchase.

Briefs are characterized by fast, global electronic dissemination, standard publishing contracts, easy-to-use manuscript preparation and formatting guidelines, and expedited production schedules. We aim for publication 8–12 weeks after acceptance.

André Pereira Neto

Strategies to Fight Online Health Misinformation

Health Information Quality Assurance, Digital Literacy and Fact-Checking

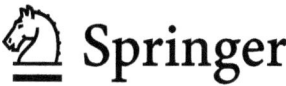

André Pereira Neto
National School of Public Health
Oswaldo Cruz Foundation
Rio de Janeiro, Rio de Janeiro, Brazil

ISSN 2192-3698　　　　　　　ISSN 2192-3701　(electronic)
SpringerBriefs in Public Health
ISBN 978-3-032-02155-7　　　ISBN 978-3-032-02156-4　(eBook)
https://doi.org/10.1007/978-3-032-02156-4

© The Editor(s) (if applicable) and The Author(s), under exclusive license to Springer Nature Switzerland AG 2025

This work is subject to copyright. All rights are solely and exclusively licensed by the Publisher, whether the whole or part of the material is concerned, specifically the rights of reprinting, reuse of illustrations, recitation, broadcasting, reproduction on microfilms or in any other physical way, and transmission or information storage and retrieval, electronic adaptation, computer software, or by similar or dissimilar methodology now known or hereafter developed.
The use of general descriptive names, registered names, trademarks, service marks, etc. in this publication does not imply, even in the absence of a specific statement, that such names are exempt from the relevant protective laws and regulations and therefore free for general use.
The publisher, the authors and the editors are safe to assume that the advice and information in this book are believed to be true and accurate at the date of publication. Neither the publisher nor the authors or the editors give a warranty, expressed or implied, with respect to the material contained herein or for any errors or omissions that may have been made. The publisher remains neutral with regard to jurisdictional claims in published maps and institutional affiliations.

This Springer imprint is published by the registered company Springer Nature Switzerland AG
The registered company address is: Gewerbestrasse 11, 6330 Cham, Switzerland

If disposing of this product, please recycle the paper.

To Miguel, my beloved grandson
This book was originally written in Portuguese. It was translated into English by MARTIM CARDOSO

Contents

1	**Digital Media, Disinformation, and Health: An Introduction**	1
	1.1 Information Society	1
	1.2 New Information and Communication Technologies: Virtues	7
	1.3 New Information and Communication Technologies: Problems	9
	1.4 New Information and Communication Technologies: Virtues in Health	15
	1.5 Infodemic and Infodemiology: Consequences and Reactions	17
	1.6 The Purpose of This Publication	19
	References	21
2	**Good Quality Health Information on the Internet: An Alternative to Combat Misinformation**	25
	2.1 The "Expert Patient" and Quality of Information	27
	2.2 Evaluation Methods	28
	2.3 Our Assessment Experience: Brief History	34
	2.4 Final Considerations	49
	References	53
3	**Digital Literacy Against Disinformation: Vital Pedagogical Practice for All of Us, Forever**	59
	3.1 Introduction	59
	3.2 Digital Exclusion	62
	3.3 Digital Literacy and the Fight Against Disinformation	68
	3.4 Digital Literacy Against Disinformation: A Vital Pedagogical Practice for All, Forever	73
	References	76
4	***Fact-Checking*: Necessary and Urgent**	79
	4.1 Introduction	79
	4.2 Fact-Checking in the World	86
	4.3 Fact-Checking Methods	88

	4.4	The Financing of Fact-Checking Agencies	91
	4.5	Last Question	94
	4.6	Final Considerations	98
	References		99
Index			103

About the Author

André Pereira Neto (PhD, 1997) is a professor of Health Information and Communication at the Oswaldo Cruz Foundation (FIOCRUZ), Rio de Janeiro, Brazil. He is one of the editors of the book "The Internet and Health in Brazil: Challenges and Trends" (Springer, 2019). He was a visiting researcher at the "Ecole des Hautes Études en Sciences de l'information et de La Communication/Sorbonne" Université, in Paris, France (2022), and at "DigiMedia - Digital Media and Interaction Research Center", in Aveiro, Portugal (2023).

Chapter 1
Digital Media, Disinformation, and Health: An Introduction

Abstract This chapter is an introduction to the book *Strategies to Fight Online Health Misinformation: Health Information Quality Assurance, Digital Literacy and Fact-Checking*. This chapter presents and analyzes the virtues and problems inherent to the "Network Society," characterized by the pervasive presence of new information and communication technologies in the lives of each of us. It highlights the interface between this context and health. It discusses the concepts of "fake news" and "disinformation." It analyzes the consequences and reactions to the information epidemic we live in ("Infodemic"), particularly in the context of COVID-19. This introduction presents, finally, the three chapters coming next in the book, where an analysis is made of alternatives to fight "misinformation," namely: health information quality assurance, digital literacy, and fact-checking. As far as we see, these alternatives should be part of public policies meant to promote citizenship against disinformation.

Keywords Networked society · Pandemic · COVID-19 · Information and communication technologies · Disinformation · Fake news · Infodemic · Infodemiology

1.1 Information Society

Economic, social, and cultural relations seem to have been transformed over the past 50 years. I refer to the increasingly pervasive and ubiquitous entry of new information and communication technologies into the lives of each of us.

The rapid introduction and wide dissemination of new information and communication technologies (ICT) in contemporary society have raised numerous topics and problems of great interest. Among them is the question of whether there has been a change and whether or not we are living in a society governed by singular rules, different from those that guided social organization until then.

In our view, this metamorphosis seems evident.

However, sometimes, immersed in this context of transformation, we do not realize its speed, intensity, and capillarity. Different observers and analysts of reality have been trying to understand this scenario in different ways for some time.

The Brazilian songwriter Gilberto Gil was one of them. In 1969, Gil recorded the song "Cérebro Eletrônico" (Electronic Brain). For Gil, in his poetic lyrics, the human being is the only one capable of performing the activities that determine the functioning of the "Electronic Brain," such as talking and walking. The poet thus admitted that the "Electronic Brain" cannot think.

For Moreira and Massarani (2006), songs have always been an important reference on culture, revealing visions, representations, and attitudes of man towards the world, life, and society. In this sense, this song by Gil can be an example of such. This songwriter did not follow the methodological rigor of the social sciences but expressed a concern present in many of us who witnessed this change closely in the late 1960s. Those who lived at that time would have difficulty admitting that we would, 50 years later, experience a reality like the one we are currently witnessing.

At the same time that Gil released his music, many social scientists, in different parts of the planet, tried to understand the changes that were taking place in society. Some of them even came out with the expression "Information Society." In this case, they sought to highlight the decisive role that information would play in the near future, in the most different fields of knowledge and production.

One of them was Daniel Bell (1919–2011). He is considered one of the pioneers in the elaboration of the expression "Information Society." Bell's (1973) ideas are based on the view that, in the mid-1970s, we would be entering a "Post-Industrial Society." It would succeed the "Industrial Society" that came to succeed the "Agrarian Society." In the "Post-Industrial Society," services would play a central role in the economy and social life. For Bell (1973), whoever managed to control the most amount of information would have more power. According to him, the domain of information would become noticeable in all economic areas, including traditional ones such as agriculture and industry. The author points out that information would have speed, flexibility, and efficiency unprecedented in human history. In addition, information would contribute to the reduction of labor costs within the capitalist logic and would cause a restructuring of the productive base.

Bell's ideas (1973) were published long before we came across the countless possibilities that new information and communication technologies provide us today. His ideas predict the existence of the robot that came to perform functions hitherto performed by man. They predate the production restructuring we now experience by means of which workers are being replaced by tools controlled by information and communication technologies.

It should be noted that Bell (1973) was not the only author who made an effort, since the middle of the last century, to understand the character of the changes that were taking place in society. Yoneji Masuda (1905–1995) also produced premonitory knowledge in this regard.

In his book *The Information Society as Post-Industrial Society*, published in 1980, Masuda (1980) emphasizes the "silent social change" that information would be promoting in society. His vision is similar to that expressed by Bell (1973), as he associates this transformation with the organization of a "Post-Industrial" society, which would be replacing the "Industrial Society," which in turn would be replacing the "Agrarian Society." According to Masuda (1980), in the "Information Society," science would play a decisive role in the production process. In Masuda's work (Masuda, 1980), the rise and prominence of professional, scientific, and technical groups would be observed, in addition to the introduction of what we now call "information and communication technologies." Another aspect worth noting, in the ideas of Masuda (1980), refers to the realm of privacy that, in his view, would tend to disappear. He speculated that people in the "Information Society" would share their personal information to create synergies and solve personal, economic, and social problems. This information would become very valuable.

Duff and Itō (2020) analyzed the work of Masuda (1980) and concluded that:

> However, broadly speaking, they all remain sound propositions. The future will be comprehensively computerized, that we know, and the human requirements of the nascent global information society are precisely what Masuda enthused about: post-materialism, information utilities, voluntary communities, time-value, and a global civic consciousness. Each of these goals is highly desirable in its own right, and could and should be sought independently. (Duff & Itō, 2020, p. 68–69)

Alvin Toffler (1928–2016) was another intellectual who had concerns similar to those expressed in the published works of Bell (1919–2011) and Masuda (1905–1995).

His first book *Future Shock* was published in 1970 in the United States. In it, Toffler (1970) makes reflections of a historical-political-economic nature and proposes to build a transdisciplinary paradigm about the directions that civilization would follow in the near future. Leaving claims and utopias aside, this book has sold more than 6 million copies and has been published in different languages.

Years later, Toffler (1928–2016) released the book *The Third Wave* (1980). In this case, the author uses the metaphor of "waves" to refer to the conflicts and tensions of each moment of change. The author clarifies, in the introduction to his book, the limitations of this metaphor but uses it to refer to the respective social, political, and economic environments that involve family, religion, and the State and that have changed over time. Toffler's (1980) ideas are close to those of Bell (1919–2011), and Masuda (1905–1995) in the way they also divide the history of humanity into watertight periods with their own characteristics.

The studies by Bell (1973), Masuda (1980) and Toffler (1970, 1980) divided history into consecutive, watertight moments based on events held in European countries.

The songwriter Gilberto Gil, with his sensitivity and creativity, announced a change where the "Electronic Brain" would command everything, or almost everything. A transformation that, according to him, was about to happen. A voice coming from the southern part of the planet anticipating, in a poetic way, a way of living that would be different from what we had been used to until then.

The views of these three intellectuals and this poet seem surprising to us, above all, because they were published a few years before the development of the "Network

Society." Premonitory as they were, these authors and this poet indicated the path being followed by capitalist society at the time.

In 1991, Dutch researcher Jan van Dijk (born in 1952) made famous the expression "Network Society" when launching his book, originally published in Dutch: *De Netwerkmaatschappij, sociale aspecten van nieuwe media* (Van Dijk, 1991). Eight years later, the same book was published in English and entitled: *The Network Society, Social Aspects of New Media* (Van Dijk, 1999).

At the same time, Castells (1996) released the book *The Rise of the Network Society*, the first volume of the trilogy *The Information Age*. This term took on unique contours in the work of the Spanish researcher.

For Castells (1996), the "Network Society" is a term that seeks to designate a society organized based on a communication system mediated by information and communication technologies that integrate a system of human interactions (economic, social, cultural, political, and behavioral) carried out in cyberspace.

Pierre Lévy, born in Tunisia in 1956, is another thinker who produced innovative and premonitory knowledge not to be forgotten. His first book on the subject, published in French, was called *La machine univers: création, cognition et culture informatique* (Lévy, 1987). In it, the author addresses some cultural implications of computerization and its roots in the history of the West. Three years later, he published, in French, the book *Les technologies de l'intelligence: L'Avenir de la pensée à l'ère informatique* (Lévy, 1990). In this case, the author remains concerned with the cultural dimension of the media phenomenon that was being announced.

In the following years, his academic production began to focus on what he called *Les arbres de connaissances* (Authier & Lévy, 1993), *L'intelligence collective: Pour une anthropologie du cyberespace* (Lévy, 1994), and finally *Cyberculture* (Lévy, 1997). In his view, cyberculture would create new ways of producing and distributing knowledge. They would bring together material and intellectual techniques, behaviors, and ways of thinking and values that develop simultaneously in cyberspace. In this sense, according to Lévy (1997), cyberculture is synonymous with change.

According to Bennis (2024):

> Cyberculture defines the social and communication structures of organizations and institutions that have adapted to the new digital environment. In this sense, cyberculture has become part and parcel of the daily life of societies, communities, and individuals. Cyberculture encompasses the key elements involved in the practice of digital culture, such as virtual communities, online identities, social media, e-commerce, online education, cyberclass. (Bennis, 2024, p. 37)

Lévy (1997) highlights in his work the role of cyberculture in the constitution of the "collective ecology," made of individuals, institutions, and techniques and dynamics populated by active singularities and changing subjectivities. His premonitory thinking came before the advent and consolidation of Web 2.0.

Web 2.0 was the second generation of the World Wide Web. It was characterized by creating the conditions for the exchange of information and collaboration between users of websites and virtual services. It was made popular in 2004 by the American company O'Reilly Media. Web 2.0 communities began to be activated through the use of collaborative applications and information-gathering tools such as wikis, blogs, forums, aggregation, instant messaging, and interactive voice. Web 2.0 enabled levels and patterns of interaction, sharing, and opinion exchange that until recently were only possible offline.

The works by Lévy (1987, 1990, 1994, 1997), van Dijk (1991, 1999), and Castells (1996) were published in the late 1980s and early 1990s. At that time, the Internet was beginning to gain popularity and interfere with citizens' privacy and their notions of time and space.

For van Dijk (1991), the "Network Society" would replace the "Mass Society," configuring itself, in his words, "a new media" (Van Dijk, 1991). For him, in the "Network Society," social relations would be organized through digital media that would complement or replace face-to-face media. They would be the "nervous system" of society. In his view, a pattern of social relationships mediated by computers (CMCs—computer-mediated communications) was being established. For van Dijk (1991), in the "Network Society," individuals would be constantly connected to each other within the digital environment. In his view, people would become increasingly dependent on these technologies. For Schumann (2013), optimism in the face of the changes that were being announced seems to characterize the ideals of this intellectual.

Castells' (1996) view differs somewhat from that presented by Van Dijk (1991). For Castells (1996), technology is shaped by society and not the other way around. For him, information and communication technologies meet the basic needs of society and the process of globalization that we have been experiencing since the middle of the last century. The new social division of labor can be considered an example in this regard. In this case, the fragmentation of the production process would be leading to the creation of various levels of specialization carried out in different parts of the planet. The new information and communication technologies facilitate the organization of the "Information Capitalism" that is at the service of globalization.

Kizilhan and Kizilhan (2016), when analyzing Castells' work, state:

> Castells mentions about Information Technology Revolution's effects on globalization, as a form of reorganization of the capitalist system within the framework of production, experience and power relations. He conceptualizes this new economic system as "Informational Capitalism". [...] According to Castells, the core of the transformation of this revolution is the information and communication technologies; and new information technologies aren't just application tools but at the same time they are processes to be developed. (Kizilhan & Kizilhan, 2016, p. 277–278).

Castells (1996) understands that the "Network Society" allows individuals or smaller groups of people to gather online and share, sell, and exchange goods, services, and information. It also enables more people, groups, and organizations to have a voice in their community and in the world at large. It integrates different media that work interactively, governed by a digital code. There is no sender or receiver anymore. Subjects are autonomous and content producers. Interactivity, without mediation, facilitates the strengthening of network sociability and the formation of *online* communities. According to him, the "Network Society" stands out for its ability to facilitate collective grouping, content production, and the wide dissemination and sharing of information. In addition, it can have a huge impact on society, both at the individual level and in the forms of social organization. The Internet is becoming an essential means of communication and organization in all spheres of activity. According to Castells, social movements and the political process use it, and will increasingly do so, as a privileged instrument to act, inform, recruit, organize, dominate, and counter-dominate.

Duff (2022) compared the ideas of Bell and Castells and admits that:

> [...] both plausibly explain contemporary social reality in terms of the interplay of three forces: the information technology revolution, the restructuring of capitalism and the innovational role of culture. There are found to be major similarities in their accounts [...] but also significant divergences (role of science, the fourth world, the normative content of culture). (Duff, 2022, p. 90)

The same "three forces" can be observed in cloud computing, Smart Cities (CIs), applications, advanced robotics, big data, artificial intelligence (AI), three-dimensional printing, virtual reality, and biotechnology (João et al., 2019). They can also be identified in the "Internet *of* Things" (IOT), the "Internet of Everything" (IOE), and the "Internet *of nano* Things" (IoNT) (Miraz et al., 2015).

Korteling et al. (2021) compare human and electronic intelligences and concluded that:

> In contrast, biology does a lot with a little: organic brains are millions of times more efficient in energy consumption than computers. The human brain consumes less energy than a lightbulb, whereas a supercomputer with comparable computational performance uses enough electricity to power quite a village [...] (Korteling et al., 2021, p. 5).

Reiterating the prophecies made by Gilberto Gil in 1969, this new "electronic brain" does everything, or almost everything, but "it does not walk." The poet highlighted in his song that only the user thinks and can decide whether to live or die. The "electronic brain" does not have this power or this ability. In addition, he admits that "only I can cry when I'm sad." It seems as if these assumptions are not evident any longer, given the unpredictable consequences of Artificial Intelligence.

Yuval Harari has just launched his book *Nexus: A Brief History of Information Networks from the Stone Age to AI* (2024). In an interview on a Brazilian TV show, Harari argues that Artificial Intelligence (AI) is fundamentally different from any previous technology in history. He claims it is the first technology capable of autonomously making decisions and generating new ideas. AI is not a mere tool. It is an independent agent. Harari compares AI to the atomic bomb! According to him, the bomb doesn't decide where to explode or who to attack. For him, AI is far more powerful because it can make such decisions, particularly in systems like autonomous weapons—deciding targets and attack locations—and can invent new weapons and strategies. Consequently, he concludes that AI, in this sense, is taking power away from humans.

The purpose of this chapter is not to analyze in detail the three forces or to evaluate the different new forms and dimensions that the new information communication technologies are taking in the life of each of us.

This brief introduction aimed to demonstrate that we live in a capitalist society governed by unique rules, different from those that guided economic organization until then. The big companies that owned land or industry are not as powerful as they once were. The richest and most powerful are those who master information. As Bell (1973) prophesied, whoever can control the greatest amount of information will have the most power and capital. The CompaniesMarketcap.com website in May 2024 (Companies Market Cap, 2024) indicates that five of the ten most profitable companies in the world operate in the area of new information and communication technologies, namely: Microsoft, Apple, Google, Amazon, and Facebook.

This "Network Society" has virtues and problems that will be presented below.

1.2 New Information and Communication Technologies: Virtues

In the "Network Society," *new* information and communication technologies (NICTs) prevail. In our view, these technologies are *new* for some distinct and complementary reasons.

On the one hand, through them, the citizen has access to an immeasurable universe of information. In traditional information and communication technologies, such as press, radio, and television, the amount of information was, and continues to be, finite. In addition, with the NICTs, this same citizen became the subject of the informational process, as it is he who decides the information he intends to obtain. In traditional media, it is the sender who defines what, when, and how the information will reach the citizen. In addition, in NICTs, the citizen, having mastered certain skills, is able to produce and share information that can "go viral" as it spreads in a way that creates a virus-like effect.

The violent murder of a Black man committed by the police in the streets of the United States had a strong repercussion on the media and unleashed a wave of protest all over the world.

George Floyd was murdered on May 25, 2020, after a Minneapolis (USA) police officer kneeled on his neck for 8 min and 46 s when he was lying face down on the street. While moaning and sobbing, he managed to utter the following sentence: "I can't breathe!". In a few moments, a video shot on a smartphone went viral and mobilized hearts and minds all over the world. The four police officers involved were terminated on the following day (NBC News, 2020).

On traditional media, production and dissemination costs prevent a citizen with few resources from disseminating their information. In this case, there is no content cluster or dependence on an advertising budget. The product is customizable and multidirectional, aimed at certain niches that translate specific interests.

This change became even more noticeable after these features migrated to the mobile device that became the smartphone (Pereira Neto & Flynn, 2019).

In recent years, there has been a substantial increase in speed, flexibility, and efficiency in the processing of information that has been accompanied by a remarkable reduction in component costs. This change has far-reaching actual and potential effects and countless cultural and social consequences.

The NICTs, with their characteristics, can serve objectively to meet the Sustainable Development Goals proposed by the United Nations in 2020 (Wu et al., 2018). Connectivity can, for example, increase productivity and competitiveness among small and medium-sized enterprises and contribute to building a more socially inclusive society by opening up new opportunities for creative and innovative work in the virtual environment. Through digital media, health services can reach many people who would have difficulty accessing them otherwise.

The virtues of the "Network Society" can also be identified in the health field.

1.2.1 New Information and Communication Technologies: Virtues in Health

What do you do when you want to know something about health or disease? Buy a newspaper or a magazine? Turn on the radio or television? Look for a healthcare professional? No! You access a search engine on your computer or smartphone and try to find the information you are looking for on the Internet. The search for health information online has become an important, unprecedented, and common resource for individuals to meet their information needs. The convenience and speed of access to a wide variety of resources and sources of information have contributed to online research taking a prominent and unique place in this context (Barbosa et al., 2023). We say unprecedented and unique because a few years ago, the reality was quite different. Those of us who write and do research often visit libraries and buy books. Until recently, going to the library meant taking a means of transport and physically entering an environment full of books. Buying a book meant going to a bookstore and looking for a book that was often not on the shelves. Now everything is at our disposal at the distance of a touch on the screen of a smartphone.

Searching and sharing information is a behavior increasingly common in most people who have access to the Internet and the skill in handling new information and communication technologies. In addition, some patients, caregivers, and other stakeholders participate in virtual patient communities to exchange information, experiences, and knowledge about different aspects related to a given disease (Barbosa & Pereira Neto, 2022).

In an online survey on the most accessed sources of information about COVID-19, Ho et al. (2020) came to the conclusion that:

> The most common sources of information related to Covid-19 were internet media (80.52%), traditional media (52.62%), family (24.36%), co-workers (23.57%), friends (21.08%), academic courses (20.18%) and medical staff (19.03%) (Ho et al., 2020, p. 3).

Access to quality online information can have another positive consequence. It can have an effect on the cost of health services (Spoelman et al., 2016). This study came to the conclusion that:

> Healthcare usage decreased by 12% after providing high-quality evidence-based online health information. These findings show that e-Health can be effective to improve self-management and reduce healthcare usage in times of increasing healthcare costs. (Spoelman et al., 2016, p. 1)

Lagan et al. (2011) carried out an investigation into identifying the impact of the internet on the decision-making process during pregnancy and concluded that information obtained on the internet can have "a visible impact on women's decision making in regards to all aspects of their pregnancy" (Lagan et al., 2011, p. 336).

Eysenbach (2001) published an article that became an international reference. In it, the expression *e-health* was coined, which, according to him, transcends the technological dimension. For him, it is an "emerging field" (Eysenbach, 2001, p. 1) characterized by the intersection of different domains, practices, and knowledge, such as medical information technology, public health, and administration. In his words, some "challenges" should be faced in different dimensions:

> These "new" challenges for the health care information technology industry were mainly (1) the ability of consumers to interact with their systems online (B2C = "business to consumer"); (2) improved possibilities for institution-to-institution transmissions of data (B2B = "business to business"); (3) new possibilities for peer-to-peer communication of consumers (C2C = "consumer to consumer"). (Eysenbach, 2001, p. 1)

Currently, on the World Health Organization website, the following definition of "Digital Health" is found:

> Digital health is the field of knowledge and practice associated with the development and use of digital technologies to improve health. Digital health expands the concept of eHealth to include digital consumers, with a wider range of smart devices and connected equipment. The following areas are commonly understood as being part of, or related to, digital health: artificial intelligence, big data, blockchain, health data, health information systems, the infodemic, the Internet of Things, interoperability and telemedicine. (World Health Organization, 2024).

The presence of new information and communication technologies in the lives of all of us has also brought countless problems, among which we highlight the digital divide, the loss of privacy, and the spread of disinformation with the false information that comes along.

1.3 New Information and Communication Technologies: Problems

Let us start by looking at privacy.

Regarding privacy, it is always good to remember that in today's society, information is the main economic asset. The information we offer for free on digital media becomes commodities that generate skyrocketing profits for a few free-of-charge platforms like Facebook, WhatsApp, Instagram, and YouTube. This is because the data we make available on these platforms on a daily basis allows public and private information agencies to control our lives and know exactly where we are, what we do, what we buy, what we sell, who we interact with, and what we think.

The invasion of privacy has become even more evident in some recent cases.

One of them involved Edward Snowden and was made public in the documentary *Citizenfour* (Poitras, 2014). He revealed in detail how our privacy is not being respected.

Bauman et al. (2015) consider that Snowden's revelations about mass surveillance had substantial political repercussions in 2013 and 2014, but also raised profound legal questions. According to the authors:

> Two distinct but interlinked Human Rights issues arise with regard to mass surveillance. The first—although it is the most fundamental and also the most often ignored—is the right of each person to have their private and family life respected. The second—generally the subject of greater political and media noise—is the duty of States to protect personal data (Bauman et al., 2015, p. 20).

Each of us realizes on a daily basis that we are being watched. Many do not care who is watching and what the purpose of this activity is. Cameras are scattered everywhere, on almost every corner. They don't hide them. They announce their presence. Their purpose is not only to regulate our behavior, as in the case of cameras placed near traffic lights, so fines can be charged for crossing the red light. They also watch over everyone's lives and are able to identify our preferences and unravel the intimate life of each of us. They are everywhere: on the street, in shopping malls, schools, airports, buildings, and vehicles. All these surveillance procedures are accepted. They are recognized as normal.

Other cases may exemplify how some information agencies invade our privacy on a daily basis and obtain information and data from each of us. One of the examples was related to the *Facebook-Cambridge Analytica scandal*. The documentary *The Great Hack* (Amer & Noujaim, 2019) reveals how *Facebook* improperly obtained data from 87 million Facebook user profiles. This scandal was not enough to change the behavior of the users of this platform.

Hinds et al. (2020) interviewed 30 students at a UK university to learn about their perception of online privacy in the wake of the scandal. They concluded that, contrary to expectations, respondents did not delete their Facebook accounts, change their privacy settings, or even express as much concern about the case as might have been expected. Many consider themselves immune to these privacy invasion strategies and do not understand how automated approaches and algorithms work in relation to their personal data.

The film *The Social Dilemma* (Orlowski, 2020) seems to be an important recommendation for reflection on the dangers and challenges that lie ahead of us. Du (2022), analyzing this film, concluded that:

> Technology can be an emancipatory, democratizing tool, capable of empowering individuals to achieve their goals and fulfill their dreams. Facebook's mission is to "give people the

1.3 New Information and Communication Technologies: Problems

power to build community and bring the world closer together." Google's is to "organize the world's information and make it universally accessible and useful." The best thing is—these services are free. Or are they really free? The Social Dilemma pulls back the curtain of big tech's lofty missions and free services to reveal an exploitative profit-maximization machine that is getting more and more powerful. (Du, 2022, p. 213)

The case involving Julian Assange is also worth mentioning.

He founded the website WikiLeaks (2006) and gained international attention in 2010 when the website published a series of thousands of confidential documents from the US government. His action had enormous repercussions and international recognition, even receiving several awards, such as the one from Amnesty International UK. Media Awards (2009). In September 2010, Assange was named one of the 50 most influential figures by the *New Statesman*, a British political magazine. Following the 2010 leaks, US authorities launched a criminal investigation into WikiLeaks, followed by a relentless persecution that sparked reactions around the world. He was imprisoned in 2010 in the United Kingdom. In 2024, he was tried and sentenced to 62 months in prison. After serving his sentence, he took refuge in the Northern Mariana Islands, near Australia, his home country.

Touchton et al. (2020) evaluate the WikiLeaks case as follows:

> The release of classified documents through outlets like WikiLeaks has transformed American politics by shedding light on the innerworkings of governments, parties, and corporations. The high-profile criminal cases associated with such releases […] have highlighted important questions about journalism, government secrecy, and the public's "right to know". (Touchton et al., 2020, p. 1)

> While the term whistleblowing tends to refer to exposures made in the public interest, a new form of exposure has come about that involves the capture and digital release of large caches of sensitive documents […]. For example, the organization WikiLeaks bypasses governments, solicits illicit materials, and releases millions of documents online […]. Such activities challenge traditional conceptions of both whistleblowing and leaking. (Touchton et al., 2020, p. 1–2)

Another negative consequence is related to the flood of misinformation.

1.3.1 Fake News or Misinformation?

As we mentioned earlier, the *New* Information and Communication Technologies have an important advantage: Anyone with access to the internet and sufficient expertise can post and share information, at any time and place, at a very low price. This information can reach thousands of people in a few seconds through online social networks. This practice generates an increasingly frequent problem: fake news. This will be the topic and issue we will look at next.

The Italian philosopher Umberto Eco (1932–2016) argues that social media has fundamentally changed public discourse by granting an equal platform to everyone. He contends that individuals whose opinions were previously confined to insignificant private settings (like bars) can now broadcast their views widely. This creates an "invasion" where such voices hold the same weight as highly respected figures (like Nobel Prize winners), which Eco views negatively. (Nicoletti, 2015).

In our view, Umberto Eco is right. However, the problem is not only the *imbeciles* who, thanks to the ease mentioned above, manage to viralize their messages. The issue also lies in the users and followers of people who make similar posts. They believe these *imbecilities* to be true. Online social media has become *what the table at the bar* used to be. Some people are sometimes suspicious of the information they receive. There are, however, those who believe *imbecile* information because it confirms their pre-established beliefs. For Eco, in the "Age of the Internet," the "conspiracy syndrome" and "rumors" are what proliferate and spread.

It is worth mentioning that cases of dissemination of imbecilities in the media are not an exclusive asset of the Internet. On the contrary, they have been present since the first writing systems, being mainly motivated by financial or ideological reasons, especially after the second half of the last century, when there was a concentration of the media in the hands of a few large companies. However, NICTs have facilitated the creation and dissemination of inaccurate and misleading information, which has come to be generically designated as *Fake News*.

In Brazil and in several parts of the world, this problem has reached the courts. It has become a matter of justice, police, and politics.

In September 2023, the Federal Supreme Court (STF) of Brazil organized the first seminar focused on the debate on "Fighting Disinformation and Defending Democracy." At the time, the Vice-President of the Court, Justice Luís Roberto Barroso, said:

> Disinformation, hate speech, murders of reputation, and conspiracy theories circulating on the internet and social media have become serious threats to democracy and to people's fundamental rights. [...] *Fakenews* have been used as an instrument of political extremism by exacerbating political polarization, fostering intolerance and, ultimately, violence. (Supremo Tribunal Federal, 2023)

Facing the "fake news" is one of the main contemporary challenges.

The definition of this expression represents a first step to be taken so that we are prepared to fight it. If we go to the Cambridge Dictionary, we will find the following meaning for *fake news*:

> false stories that appear to be news, spread on the internet or using other media, usually created to influence political views or as a joke. (Cambridge Dictionary, 2019)

In the Portuguese Online Dictionary, there is a distinct meaning, namely:

> Fake news or false information that is shared as if it were real and true, disseminated in virtual contexts, especially on social networks or in message-sharing applications. (Dicionário Online de Português, 2024, translated by the author)

The same dictionary finishes this definition by stating that:

> The term *Fake News*, although widely used, has not yet been formally integrated into the list of words in the Portuguese language, so it is a foreignism. (Dicionário Online de Português, 2024, translated by the author)

1.3 New Information and Communication Technologies: Problems

Wardle and Derakhshan (2017) published a report under the auspices of the European Community on the subject. According to Google Scholar, by May 2024, this report had been cited 2970 times. We can admit, therefore, that it has become an important international reference in the debate.

In the synopsis of this report, the authors state that:

> […] we are witnessing something new: information pollution at a global scale; a complex web of motivations for creating, disseminating and consuming these 'polluted' messages; a myriad of content types and techniques for amplifying content; innumerable platforms hosting and reproducing this content; and breakneck speeds of communication between trusted peers. (Wardle & Derakhshan, 2017, p. 4)

They admit, in the introduction to the same report, that the emergence of the Internet and online social networks has brought about fundamental changes in the way information is produced, communicated, and distributed. They identify the following characteristics of information on online social networks, namely:

> a) Widely accessible, cheap and sophisticated editing and publishing technology has made it easier than ever for anyone to create and distribute content; b) Information consumption, which was once private, has become public because of social media; c) The speed at which information is disseminated has been supercharged by an accelerated news cycle and mobile handsets; d) Information is passed in real-time between trusted peers, and any piece of information is far less likely to be challenged. (Wardle & Derakhshan, 2017, p. 11–12).

For them, "information pollution" has direct and indirect impacts that are difficult to quantify. They start the report by condemning the use of the expression *fake news* for a few reasons:

> First, it is woefully inadequate to describe the complex phenomena of information pollution. The term has also begun to be appropriated by politicians around the world to describe news organisations whose coverage they find disagreeable. In this way, it's becoming a mechanism by which the powerful can clamp down upon, restrict, undermine and circumvent the free press. (Wardle & Derakhshan, 2017, p. 5).

We agree with the point of view of Wardle and Derakhshan (2017). In our view, the term "fake news" has become insufficient to encompass the different meanings that the social phenomenon of disinformation has recently taken on. In fact, this term has come to have different meanings varying according to the person or group using it. The plasticity and malleability of the word "fake news" lacked an expression that better translated its different dimensions.

Wardle and Derakhshan (2017) propose, in this report, that the word "fake news" be replaced by three expressions of disinformation: "misinformation, disinformation, and malinformation." They drew a distinction between these three expressions "using the dimensions of harm and falseness":

> *Mis-information* is when false information is shared, but no harm is meant.
> *Dis-information* is when false information is knowingly shared to cause harm.
> *Mal-information* is when genuine information is shared to cause harm, often by moving information designed to stay private into the public sphere. (Wardle & Derakhshan, 2017, p. 5)

For Wardle and Derakhshan (2017), the act of communicating is not restricted to transmitting information from one person to another. The authors insist on recognizing "that communication plays a fundamental role in representing shared beliefs" (Wardle & Derakhshan, 2017, p. 7).

Aïmeur et al. (2023) recently published a literature review whose objective was "to provide a comprehensive and systematic review of fake news research as well as a fundamental review of existing approaches used to detect and prevent fake news from spreading via Online Social Networks (OSNs)" (Aïmeur et al., 2023, p. 1).

This is a study carried out in the main international bibliographic databases in which the authors examine the academic production of the last 10 years. However, the survey indicated that production on the subject increased significantly during and after 2019. The authors read the abstracts, excluded some articles, and selected 61 titles that discuss the definition of the term "fake news" and other issues related to this debate.

The abstract of Aïmeur et al.'s (2023) article contains a brief assessment of the importance of "fake news" in the contemporary scenario.

> Online social networks (OSNs) are rapidly growing and have become a huge source of all kinds of global and local news for millions of users. However, OSNs are a double-edged sword. In spite of the great advantages they offer, such as unlimited easy communication and instant news and information, they can also have many disadvantages and issues. One of their major challenging issues is the spread of fake news. Fake news identification is still a complex unresolved issue. Furthermore, fake news detection on OSNs presents unique characteristics and challenges that make finding a solution anything but trivial (Aïmeur et al., 2023, p. 1).

One of the results of the bibliographic investigation carried out by Aïmeur et al. (2023) indicates that there is still no consensual definition of the term "fake news." One of the objectives of this study was to "identify the terms and features most commonly used to define fake news and categorize related works accordingly." They also propose to create "a fake news typology classification based on the various categorizations of fake news reported in the literature" (Aïmeur et al., 2023, p. 4).

This typology proposes three types of disinformation, namely: "Misinformation" would be false information that is shared without the intention to mislead or to cause harm. "Disinformation" would be false information that is shared to intentionally mislead. "Malinformation" would be genuine information that is shared with the intention to cause harm.

Thus, the literature review published in 2023 indicates that the three terms and their meaning, present in the text of Wardle and Derakhshan (2017), remain current.

Oliveira (2020) criticized the proposal made by Wardle and Derakhshan (2017). The author understands that this idea is based on the linear model of the field of communication, where it is possible to make a deduction on the intention of subjects.

In spite of the remarks made by Oliveira (2020), the term "disinformation" will serve as a reference for the analysis we will make in this book.

We will see below how disinformation has a negative impact on health.

1.4 New Information and Communication Technologies: Virtues in Health

Incorrect, incomprehensible, and outdated information, whether or not intended to cause harm, can have negative consequences for the health and well-being of citizens and communities. False information can harm human health. Many false or misleading stories are invented and shared without the receiver bothering to verify the quality of the source or the source itself. A lot of this false information is based on conspiracy theories. Some insert elements of these theories into a believable discourse. Every day, there is inaccurate, false, and unscientific information about different diseases that encompasses their transmission, cause, prevention, and treatment. Other incorrect information on disease prevention and health promotion is also present in digital media.

Wang et al. (2019) present the results of a systematic review on the diffusion of disinformation on digital media, focusing especially on the health field. In the abstract of this article, they state that:

> Contemporary commentators describe the current period as "an era of fake news" in which misinformation, generated intentionally or unintentionally, spreads rapidly. Although affecting all areas of life, it poses particular problems in the health arena, where it can delay or prevent effective care, in some cases threatening the lives of individuals. While examples of the rapid spread of misinformation date back to the earliest days of scientific medicine, the internet, by allowing instantaneous communication and powerful amplification has brought about a quantum change (Wang et al., 2019, p. 1).

The COVID-19 Pandemic was a fertile stage for the spread of false information. The production of investigations inventorying examples that describe and analyze the consequences of false information on health was fertile. Some emphasize the influence of disinformation on management and others on the behavior of citizens.

In the first case, it is worth highlighting the vision of Posenato and Duarte (2020) where they admit that:

> Too much information, often conflicting, makes it difficult to find those that are truly useful for guiding people, and can make it difficult for managers and health professionals to make decisions, especially when there is not enough time to evaluate the available evidence. (Posenato & Duarte, 2020, p. 1)

False information also interfered with vaccination coverage.

Galhardi et al. (2022), in a quantitative empirical study, worked with a sample of 253 checks on vaccines and COVID-19, using the "Eu Fiscalizo" application. The study pointed out that the Coronavac vaccine, produced by the Butantã Institute in partnership with the Chinese company Sinovac, was the immunizer that had the highest amount of fake news related to it. The study found that in at least 70% of Brazilian municipalities, many people, supported by xenophobic rhetoric, refused to take precisely this immunizer. This, however, was not the only justification for the rejection of vaccination. Galhardi et al. (2022) describe the different arguments that led many people not to accept vaccination with Coronavac as follows:

During the pandemic, public statements by the President of the Republic Jair Bolsonaro contributed to legitimizing vaccine hesitancy, giving greater visibility and scope to his arguments. Although articulated mainly through social networks, the hesitant individuals themselves are not a homogeneous group. They may refuse only one or several vaccines for several reasons, among which are the beliefs that a) The vaccine contains toxic elements; b) the child's immune system is immature to deal with so many vaccines; c) vaccines are part of a commercial conspiracy by the pharmaceutical industry; d) natural immunity is better; e) most diseases are harmless to most children; f) vaccine-preventable diseases were reduced by improving health conditions, and not because of vaccination; g) the release of virus by residues, after the administration of a live virus vaccine, can lead to illness. (Galhardi et al., 2022, p. 1851)

Another study associates the greater or lesser presence of digital media with the mortality rates of the disease.

Nieves-Cuervo et al. (2021) published on the website of the Pan American Health Organization the results of a research in which they sought to identify this possible association. Some cases were highlighted.

Chile and Argentina were the countries with the greatest internet penetration rates (92.4% and 92.0%, respectively) and were also among the heaviest users of social media as their only means of obtaining news (32.0% and 28.0%, respectively). (Nieves-Cuervo et al., 2021, p. 1)

Disinformation can interfere in human behavior. It can also kill!

Jolley and Paterson (2020) analyzed a phenomenon observed in Europe, North America, and Australia where information was disseminated in digital media that related 5G mobile phone technology to the spread of the new coronavirus. This study concluded that:

During the COVID-19 pandemic, telecommunication masts across Europe, North America, and Australasia have been damaged or destroyed in arson attacks, while engineers have been subjected to verbal and physical abuse. [...] According to police officials and media commentators, the perpetrators are likely to be motivated by the erroneous conspiratorial belief that electromagnetic waves transmitted by 5G technology have somehow caused COVID-19 and so respond with violent actions to stop, what they see, as the origin of COVID-19. (Jolley & Paterson, 2020, p. 628)

False information can also be associated with a lack of information.

Pereira Neto et al. (2022) analyzed the quality of information from four public websites in the State of Mato Grosso do Sul, Brazil. They concluded this study by stating that these official websites did not present essential information on procedures related to the prevention of COVID-19 transmission, such as the need to wear a mask, wash hands, and use alcohol gel. The absence of information such as this may interfere with the adoption of preventive measures.

This brief presentation seems sufficient to demonstrate that false information represents a serious public health problem. It contributes to the discredit of research institutions and scientifically based guidelines. It builds a fertile field for an environment of panic and anxiety among the population. The lack of correct, up-to-date, and understandable information ends up leading citizens to believe in fake news, with or without the intention of causing harm, which circulates freely in digital media (Braz et al., 2022).

1.5 Infodemic and Infodemiology: Consequences and Reactions

During the pandemic, the Pan American Health Organization (PAHO) released an information leaflet entitled "Understanding the infodemic and misinformation in the fight against COVID-19" (Pan American Health Organization, 2020). In it, PAHO states that the COVID-19 outbreak has been accompanied by:

> A massive infodemic: an overabundance of information—some accurate and some not— that makes it hard for people to find trustworthy sources and reliable guidance when they need it. Infodemic refers to a large increase in the volume of information associated with a specific topic and whose growth can occur exponentially in a short period of time due to a specific incident, such as the current pandemic. In this situation, misinformation and rumors appear on the scene, along with manipulation of information with doubtful intent. In the information age, this phenomenon is amplified through social networks, spreading farther and faster like a virus. (Pan American Health Organization, 2020, p. 2).

Around the same time, Sylvie Briand, director of the World Health Organization, gave a statement to *The Lancet*, saying:

> We know that every outbreak will be accompanied by a kind of tsunami of information, but also within this information you always have misinformation, rumours, etc. We know that even in the Middle Ages there was this phenomenon.
> But the difference now with social media is that this phenomenon is amplified, it goes faster and further, like the viruses that travel with people and go faster and further. So it is a new challenge, and the challenge is the [timing] because you need to be faster if you want to fill the void…What is at stake during an outbreak is making sure people will do the right thing to control the disease or to mitigate its impact. So it is not only information to make sure people are informed; it is also making sure people are informed to act appropriately. (Zarocostas, 2020, p. 1)

Twenty years earlier, Eysenbach et al. (2002) published a systematic review evaluating the quality of information present on health websites. They concluded that much of the health information available on these sites was not in line with the scientific evidence. Thus, they found the existence of "individual's risk […] of encountering an inadequate site on the Web […] and the inability of the individual (or his tools) to filter the inadequate sites" (Eysenbach et al., 2002, p. 2698).

That same year, Eysenbach et al. (2002) already used the expression "disinformation," and not fake news. In this article, he announced the existence of *infodemic* and proposed the creation of a new discipline: "infodemiology."

> A new research discipline and methodology has emerged—the study of the determinants and distribution of health information and misinformation—which may be useful in guiding health professionals and patients to quality health information on the Internet. Information epidemiology, or infodemiology, identifies areas where there is a knowledge translation gap between best evidence (what some experts know) and practice (what most people do or believe), as well as markers for "high quality" information. (Eysenbach, 2002, p. 763)

PAHO, in the same fact sheet published in 2020 (Pan American Health Organization, 2020) proposed a series of initiatives to help people in the fight against the infodemic such as: identify evidence, avoid fake news, support open science, report harmful rumors, protect privacy, participate responsibly in social conversations, share information responsibly, confirm the source, in particular the threads on WhatApp (Pan American Health Organization, 2020, p. 4).

Following these initiatives, we can conclude that the responsibility for combating disinformation lies with the user.

The World Health Organization also played its part in this fight by organizing the "WHO Information Network for Epidemics." The purpose of this network would be:

> to give everyone access to timely, accurate, and easy-to-understand advice and information from trusted sources on public health events and outbreaks—currently, the COVID-19 public health emergency (Pan American Health Organization, 2020, p. 4).

In 2022, the World Health Organization published a document establishing four central points in the management of the infodemic during COVID-19, namely:

> Train health workers […]. Tailor health, information and digital literacy initiatives […]. Strive to develop high-quality, accessible health information in different digital formats […]. Establish an infodemic workforce by training staff to fulfill these functions and […] ensure this function is clearly linked to and aligned with risk communications and community engagement efforts. (World Health Organization, 2022, p. 1).

We were living through the pandemic, and the infodemic was infecting many of us.

The PAHO website that is on the air (May 2024) contains five strategic pillars for the next 5 years of the organization, namely:

> 1. Completion of pandemic control; 2. Implementation of lessons learned during the pandemic; 3. Recovery from the impacts of the pandemic on priority health programs, returning better than we were in 2019; 4. Construction of resilient National Health Systems based on renewed and strengthened Primary Health Care; 5. Permanent modernization and improvement of PAHO's management. (Pan American Health Organization, 2024)

The infodemic seems to be off the agenda. The details of the first pillar contain the following text:

> Even when vaccines were developed, we faced unconscionable obstacles: our vast region struggled to access sufficient supplies, just as misinformation increased vaccine hesitancy. Against these barriers, PAHO has worked hard to support National Immunization Plans, reinforce the cold chain capacity, provide training for health workers, improve communication strategies, and expedite access through our Revolving Fund. (Pan American Health Organization, 2024)

In the view of PAHO's Director General, disinformation is concentrated only in resistance to vaccination.

The relative neglect in tackling the problem of health misinformation is not just the fault of policymakers like Brazilian Jarbas Barbosa, who heads PAHO.

In Brazil, the most important scientific association for public health has also taken a similar stance. At the end of 2022, mass vaccination heralded the beginning of the end of the COVID-19 pandemic: Years of terror that led to the deaths of millions of people around the world. Years in which misinformation dominated digital media.

At the end of 2022, the 13th Brazilian Congress of Public Health (ABRASCO) was held in the city of Salvador, in the state of Bahia. This event was organized by the State Secretariat of Health and Science, Technology and Innovation of Bahia, the Municipal Health Secretariat of Salvador, the Council of Municipal Health Secretaries of Bahia, the State Health Council, the Federal and State Universities of Bahia, and the Oswaldo Cruz Foundation of Bahia. The central theme of this event was: "Health is democracy: diversity, equity and social justice." The topic of misinformation was only covered in 1 of the 13 thematic axes that brought together the papers presented at this event.

Fortunately, indifference seems to be losing ground in the face of the alarming evidence that the challenge of confronting misinformation presents us with every day.

In July 2024, a call for support for research projects was launched in Brazil that aims to significantly contribute to the country's scientific and technological development and innovation in the area of health misinformation (Cnpq.br, 2024). The approved proposals will be financed with resources totaling R$10,000,000.00 (10 million reais), approximately 277 thousand dollars.

In international terms, the global campaign carried out by Health Information For All (HIFA), linked to the World Health Organization, is worth highlighting. It is a network that brings together more than 19,000 health professionals, librarians, publishers, researchers, policymakers, and human rights activists from 3000 organizations in 180 countries. This initiative is based on the following principle:

> People are dying for lack of knowledge. […] Many would still be alive today if their parent, caregiver or health worker had access to basic healthcare information. […] Citizens and healthcare providers in low-resource settings do not have access to relevant, reliable healthcare information, contributing to massive unnecessary death and suffering. (Healthcare Information For All, 2024)

Our book rescues the importance of combating the infodemic for the present day.

1.6 The Purpose of This Publication

The proposal of this publication is structured on some central ideas.

We start from the assumption that we live in an "Information Society" or in the "Network Society."

In this society, health is one of the areas where information is increasingly available and shared on digital media and social media for an increasing number of stakeholders. This information, conveyed and shared on digital media may be outdated, incomplete, incorrect, or deliberately intended to mislead interlocutors. In health, misinformation can interfere with well-being or cause harm to the individual and society. In an extreme situation, misinformation can promote disease and facilitate death. On the other hand, quality online information, with a reliable, up-to-date, scientifically based, and understandable source, can play a fundamental role in self-care practices, in reducing service costs, in disease prevention, and in health promotion. With it, professionals and users of health services can learn about and possibly adopt the preventive measures recommended by science. They will also be able to know where, when, and why to perform certain diagnostic tests and receive the possible and necessary medical care.

Three reactions have been advocated in the fight against misinformation: fact-checking, digital literacy, and offering quality information.

Fact-checking is a journalistic method through which it is possible to certify whether the information distributed was obtained through reliable sources, and also to assess whether it is true or false, and whether it is sustainable or not. Its purpose is to detect and disclose errors, inaccuracies, and lies.

Digital literacy aims to develop educational interventions for the effective use of information and communication technologies. It aims to educate users to identify sources to look for the information they need or seek, to recognize the conditions under which it was produced, and to check whether it can (or cannot) be shared.

Some institutions certify virtual environments. To this end, they award a quality seal to virtual environments that comply with their principles and criteria. Others guide users on the precautions to be taken when using these environments. In both cases, different methods, criteria, and indicators are used to assess the quality of information available on the Internet. As far as we see, public institutions and institutions of public interest have the obligation to offer quality information, in other words, scientifically based, updated, and understandable to all.

For these reasons, fact-checking, digital literacy, and certification of virtual environments are some strategies to fight misinformation in health.

This book aims to address, with clear and understandable language, the three main reactions to misinformation: fact-checking agencies, digital literacy, and providing quality health information.

This book will be based on systematic reviews on the topic and recently published studies. The following three chapters will address methodological issues and successful experiences, their limitations, and scope in the field of confronting misinformation in the world, namely: fact-checking agencies, digital literacy, and evaluating health information in virtual environments aiming to offer quality information.

The book aims to offer health professionals and users of health services a brief introduction to the three main tools available to combat different forms of misinformation in the health field. The book is not intended to teach readers how to perform tasks as fact-checkers, educators, or certifiers.

The chapters are sharpened to point to strategies that are within the mandate of health professionals and users of health services, and describe how and whether they should use them, and what downstream effects of their actions may be. The book analyzes an important topic and could be useful in medical and public health programs, as well as for practicing physicians, science communicators, and users of health services.

This book proposes that combating the infodemic should become a public policy. It should become a duty of the State and public interest institutions!

Public and public interest agencies should carry out digital literacy activities with the aim of helping users use information obtained and shared on digital media in a critical and creative way. This will enable them to discern what is true from what is doubtful and to stop consuming and sharing misinformation.

Public and public interest agencies should build serious, systematic fact-checking initiatives in different areas of knowledge and human activity, especially in the health area, where misinformation can cause serious harm. Their action should be immediate. To this end, an organization should be constantly advising and monitoring the avalanche of misinformation that plagues the digital world, especially in the health field.

Public and public interest agencies should offer clear, understandable, and scientifically updated information to everyone, regardless of their level of education. This is because quality information can alleviate pain, prevent illness, and save lives. Incorrect, outdated, or incomprehensible information can cause harm to citizens and communities.

Quality information saves lives!

References

Aïmeur, E., Amri, S., & Brassard, G. (2023). Fake news, disinformation and misinformation in social media: A review. *Social Network Analysis and Mining, 13*(30).

Amer, K., & Noujaim, J. (2019). *The great hack*. Netflix.

Authier, M., & Lévy, P. (1993). *Les arbres de connaissances*. La Découverte.

Barbosa, L., & Pereira Neto, A. (2022). Communication and information about breast cancer: A comparative study between a physical and an online environment. In G. Meiselwitz (Ed.), *Social computing and social media: Design, user experience and impact* (pp. 3–12). Springer.

Barbosa, L., Pereira Neto, A., & Felipette, J. (2023). Avaliação da qualidade da informação de saúde on-line: uma análise bibliográfica da produção acadêmica brasileira [Evaluation of the quality of online health information: a bibliographic analysis of Brazilian academic production]. *Saúde debate, 47*(137), 272–283.

Bauman, Z., Bigo, D., Esteves, P., et al. (2015). After Snowden: Rethinking the impact of surveillance. *Rev Eco-Pós, 18*(2), 8–35.

Bell, D. (1973). *The coming of Post-Industrial Society: A venture in social forecasting*. Basic Books.

Bennis, M. (2024). Cyberculture/cyberspace as a mode of transmission of cultures, identities and power relations: A theoretical perspective. *JHSSS, 6*(6), 36–42.

Braz, G., Vasconcelos, G. V. B., Amorim, E. C., et al. (2022). Fake news about COVID-19 in Brazil: An integrative review. *Diversitas Journal, 7*(1), 246–255.

Cambridge Dictionary. (2019). Fake News | Meaning in the Cambridge English Dictionary. [online]. Cambridge.org. Accessed April 28, 2025, from https://dictionary.cambridge.org/dictionary/english/fake-news

Canal GNT. (2024). *Yuval Harari fala sobre lançamento de Nexus e inteligência artificial! | Conversa Com Bial*. [online] YouTube. Accessed April 27, 2025, from https://www.youtube.com/watch?v=7kJLq2rBqRI

Castells, M. (1996). *The rise of the network society*. Blackwell.

Companies Market Cap. (2024). *Companies ranked by Market Cap*. [online] CompaniesMarketcap.com. Accessed April 27, 2025, from https://companiesmarketcap.com/

Cnpq.br. (2024). *Chamada CNPq/Decit/SECTICS/MS - N° 30/2024 - Prevenção e Enfrentamento à Desinformação Científica em Saúde - Portal CNPq*. [online] Accessed April 26, 2025, from http://memoria2.cnpq.br/web/guest/chamadas-publicas?p_p_id=resultadosportlet_WAR_resultadoscnpqportlet_INSTANCE_0ZaM&filtro=abertas&detalha=chamadaDivulgada&idDivulgacao=12405

Dicionário Online de Português. (2024). *Fake news*. [online] Dicio. Accessed April 28, 2025, from https://www.dicio.com.br/fake-news/

Du, S. (2022). Reimagining the future of technology: "The Social Dilemma" review. *Journal of Business Ethics, 177*, 213–215.

Duff, A. S. (2022). Castells versus Bell: A comparison of two grand theorists of the information age. *European Journal of Social Theory, 26*(1), 90–108.

Duff, A. S., & Itō, Y. (2020). Computopia revisited: Yoneji Masuda's realistic utopianism. *Keio communication review, 42*(3), 53–74.

Eysenbach, G. (2001). What is e-health? *Journal of Medical Internet Research, 3*(2), E20.

Eysenbach, G. (2002). Infodemiology: The epidemiology of (mis)information. *The American Journal of Medicine, 113*(9), 763–765.

Eysenbach, G., Powell, J., Kuss, O., et al. (2002). Empirical studies assessing the quality of health information for consumers on the World Wide Web: A systematic review. *JAMA, 287*(20), 2691–2700.

Galhardi, C. P., Freire, N. P., & Fagundes, M. C. M. (2022). Fake News and vaccine hesitancy in the COVID-19 pandemic in Brazil. *Ciênc Saúde Coletiva, 27*, 1849–1858.

Gil, G. (1969). *Cérebro eletrônico*. Philips. Accessed April 27, 2025, from https://www.youtube.com/watch?v=sIHG5XFPmgw

Healthcare Information For All. (2024). *Health Information For All* (HIFA.ORG). [online] Hifa.org. Accessed April 28, 2025, from https://www.hifa.org/

Hinds, J., Williams, E., & Joinson, A. (2020). "It wouldn't happen to me": Privacy concerns and perspectives following the Cambridge Analytica scandal. *International Journal of Human Computer Studies, 143*, 102498.

Ho, H., Chen, Y., & Yen, C. (2020). Different impacts of COVID-19-related information sources on public worry: An online survey through social media. *Internet Interventions, 22*, 100350.

João, B. D. N., Souza, C. L. D., & Serralvo, F. A. (2019). A systematic review of smart cities and the internet of things as a research topic. *Cad EBAPEBR, 17*, 1115–1130.

Jolley, D., & Paterson, J. L. (2020). Pylons ablaze: Examining the role of 5G COVID-19 conspiracy beliefs and support for violence. *The British Journal of Social Psychology, 59*, 628–640.

Kizilhan, T., & Kizilhan, S. B. (2016). Book Review: The rise of the network society - the information age: Economy, society, and culture. *Contemporary Educational Technology, 7*(3), 277–280.

Korteling, J. E. H., van de Boer-Visschedijk, G. C., Blankendaal, R. A. M., et al. (2021). Human versus artificial intelligence. *Frontiers in Artificial Intelligence, 4*, 622364.

Lagan, B. M., Sinclair, M., & Kernohan, W. G. (2011). What is the impact of the internet on decision-making in pregnancy? A global study. *Birth, 38*(4), 336–345.

Lévy, P. (1987). *La Machine univers: Création, cognition et culture informatique*. La Découverte.

Lévy, P. (1990). *Les technologies de l'intelligence : L'Avenir de la pensée à l'ère informatique*. La Découverte.

Lévy, P. (1994). *L'intelligence collective: Pour une anthropologie du cyberespace*. La Découverte, Paris.

Lévy, P. (1997). *Cyberculture*. Odile Jacob.

Masuda, Y. (1980). *The information as Post-Industrial Society*. Institute for the Information Society.

Miraz, M. H., Ali, M., Excell, P. S., et al. (2015). A review on Internet of Things (IoT), Internet of Everything (IoE) and Internet of Nano Things (IoNT). In: *2015 Internet Technologies and Applications (ITA) [online]. Proceedings of the Sixth International Conference (ITA 15)*,

Wrexham, UK, 2015 (pp. 219–224). Wrexham: IEEE. Accessed April 27, 2025, from https://ieeexplore.ieee.org/document/7317398/authors#authors

Moreira, I. C., & Massarani, L. (2006). (En)canto científico: temas de ciência em letras da música popular brasileira. *Hist cienc saude-Manguinhos, 13*, 291–307.

NBC News. (2020). *Watch a minute-to-minute breakdown leading up to George Floyd's deadly arrest* | NBC News NOW. YouTube. Accessed April 27, 2025, from https://www.youtube.com/watch?v=kiSm0Nuqomg

Nicoletti, G. (2015). *Umberto Eco: 'Con i social parola a legioni di imbecilli'*. [online] La Stampa. Accessed April 27, 2025, from https://www.lastampa.it/cultura/2015/06/11/news/umberto-eco-con-i-social-parola-a-legioni-di-imbecilli-1.35250428/

Nieves-Cuervo, G. M., Manrique-Hernández, E. F., Robledo-Colonia, A. F., et al. (2021). Infodemia: noticias falsas y tendencias de mortalidad por COVID-19 en seis países de América Latina [Infodemic: fake news and COVID-19 mortality trends in six Latin American countries]. *Revista Panamericana de Salud Pública, 45*, e44.

Oliveira, T. M. (2020). Como enfrentar a desinformação científica? Desafios sociais, políticos e jurídicos intensificados no contexto da pandemia. *Liinc em Revista, 16*(2), e5374.

Orlowski, J. (2020). *The social dilemma*. Netflix.

Pan American Health Organization. (2020). *Understanding the infodemic and misinformation in the fight against COVID-19*. Pan American Health Organization.

Pan American Health Organization. (2024). *Dr. Jarbas Barbosa's Vision*. [online] Paho.org. Accessed April 27, 2025, from https://www.paho.org/en/dr-jarbas-barbosas-vision

Pereira Neto, A., Ferreira, E. C., & Domingos, R. L. A. M. T. (2022). Evaluation of the quality of information on Covid-19 websites: An alternative to combat fake news. *Saúde debate, 46*(132), 30–46.

Pereira Neto, A., & Flynn, M. B. (2019). The internet and health in Brazil: Trends and challenges. In A. Pereira Neto & M. Flynn (Eds.), *The internet and health in Brazil* (pp. 1–11). Springer.

Poitras, L. (2014). *Citizenfour*. HBO Documentary Films.

Posenato, L., & Duarte, E. (2020). Infodemia: excesso de quantidade em detrimento da qualidade das informações sobre a COVID-19. *Epidemiol Serv Saúde, 29*(4), e2020186.

Schumann, S. (2013). Jan Van Dijk: The Network Society. London: Sage Publications. 2012. *MedieKultur: Journal of Media and Communication Research, 29*(54), 189–192.

Spoelman, W. A., Bonten, T. N., Waal, M. W., et al. (2016). Effect of an evidence-based website on healthcare usage: An interrupted time-series study. *BMJ Open, 6*(11), e013166.

Supremo Tribunal Federal. (2023). *Painel no Seminário de combate à desinformação discute medidas para fortalecer o sistema de Justiça*. [online] Supremo Tribunal Federal. Accessed April 27, 2025, from https://portal.stf.jus.br/noticias/verNoticiaDetalhe.asp?idConteudo=514078&ori=1

Touchton, M. R., Klofstad, C. A., West, J. P., et al. (2020). Whistleblowing or leaking? Public opinion toward Assange, Manning, and Snowden. *Research & Politics, 7*(1), 2053168020904582.

Toffler, A. (1970). *Future Schock*. Bantam Books.

Toffler, A. (1980). *The third wave: The classic study of tomorrow*. Bantam Books.

Van Dijk, J. (1991). *De netwerkmaatschappij : sociale aspecten van nieuwe media*. Bohn Stafleu Van Loghum.

Van Dijk, J. (1999). *The Network Society: Social aspects of new media*. Sage.

Wang, Y., McKee, M., Torbica, A., et al. (2019). Systematic literature review on the spread of health-related misinformation on social media. *Social Science & Medicine, 240*, 112552.

Wardle, C., & Derakhshan, H. (2017). *Information disorder: Toward an interdisciplinary framework for research and policymaking*. Council of Europe.

World Health Organization. (2022). WHO policy brief: COVID-19 infodemic management. World Health Organization. Accessed April 27, 2025, from https://www.who.int/publications/i/item/WHO-2019-nCoV-Policy_Brief-Infodemic-2022.1

World Health Organization. (2024). *Digital health.* [online] www.who.int. Accessed April 27, 2025, from https://www.who.int/europe/health-topics/digital-health#tab=tab_1

Wu, S., Guo, H., Huang, W., et al. (2018). Information and communications technologies for sustainable development goals: State-of-the-art, needs and perspectives. *IEEE Communications Surveys & Tutorials, 20*(3), 2389–2406.

Zarocostas, J. (2020). How to fight an infodemic. *The Lancet, 395*(10225), 676.

Chapter 2
Good Quality Health Information on the Internet: An Alternative to Combat Misinformation

Abstract This is the second chapter of the book *Strategies to Fight Online Health Misinformation: Health Information Quality Assurance, Digital Literacy and Fact-Checking*. It analyzes the role that the countless health information available, accessible, and shared in digital media plays in the formation of the "expert patient" and in the doctor–patient relationship. It highlights the problem of disinformation in health and analyzes different alternatives to face it, among which stands out *DISCERN*—a tool created at Oxford University. It presents the historical process of building our methodological proposal for evaluating the quality of health information on the Internet. It proposes that the indicators for evaluating the accuracy of scientific information be obtained in "summaries synthesized for clinical reference" such as *DynaMed* and not through "expert consensus." It evaluates the cases of scientific information on tuberculosis and leishmaniasis on websites, either public or of public interest, from different regions of the world. The results give evidence that some information available in these virtual environments is incorrect, outdated, or non-existent. This is a serious problem that needs to be addressed. It proposes that these institutions be committed to offering quality health information to all citizens. This is one way to encourage "expert patient" training, fight misinformation, and promote life.

Keywords Health communication · Internet · Patient portals · Disinformation · Information asymmetry · Evidence-based medicine

The interaction between New Information and Communication Technologies (NICTs) and the citizen has promoted a series of transformations that can be perceived in the way each of us carries out our daily activities.

Financial transactions, transportation, food, and education are increasingly being mediated by virtual resources. Thus, there is a growth in the number of people who: share information and knowledge through Facebook, Instagram, and WhatsApp; buy and sell products on websites such as eBay, Mercado Livre, or Amazon; commute through Uber; order food on iFood; and educate themselves with pedagogical resources available remotely, either synchronously or not. In many countries, such as Brazil, elections are held through computer terminals, and income tax is filed and sent over the Internet. If we drive and cross a red light, a camera photographs the license plate of our car, and we are then sent, by email, a copy of the photo and information on the amount of the fine. These are some examples of the presence of information accessed, produced, disseminated, and shared in digital media and directly affecting the lives of each of us.

The advantages and problems that derive from this reality were analyzed in the first chapter of this book. However, one aspect that seems relevant to us should be emphasized: information is everywhere!

Not long ago, for someone to obtain information, it was necessary to have the purchasing power to buy a newspaper or go to a library, often distant and inaccessible. Letters were sent by mail and required a certain amount of time to reach their destination. New Information and Communication Technologies (NICTs) make a myriad of information available to citizens within seconds. Much of it would not have been accessed at this same speed previously. NICTs offer unprecedented opportunities in terms of having access to information and also in having it produced and disseminated. Today, it is possible for anyone to access, produce, and share information. These skills were restricted, until recently, to certain sociocultural groups. To perform these tasks, it is necessary for the individual to have the purchasing power to acquire an electronic communication device, the socioeconomic conditions to access the network, and the skills to handle the different technological tools involved. It should be noted that the information available on the Internet is unlimited and covers any subject. This reality was compared by Pierre Lévy to a deluge: a "flood of information" (Lévy, 2001, p. XIII).

What about health on the Internet? Does this topic arouse the interest of the digital media user? Recent figures indicate that it does.

In the USA, for example, the "Center for Health Statistics" of the "National Centers for Disease Control and Prevention" of the "U.S. Department of Health and Human Services" conducted a "National Health Interview Survey" (NHIS) between July and December 2022 (Wang & Cohen, 2023). One of its results is that 58.5% of adults accessed the Internet to obtain health information. A small prevalence of women (63.3%) over men (53.5%) having this practice was identified. This number reaches 67% among adults in the 30–44 age group (Wang & Cohen, 2023).

Research published in 2021 by *EUROSTATS*—the official statistics body of the European Union—found that one in two EU citizens (55%), aged between 16 and 74, search for health information on the Internet (European Union, 2022).

In Brazil, a 2020 national survey coordinated by the "Núcleo de Informação e Coordenação do Ponto BR" of the "Comitê Gestor de Internet no Brasil" (CGI.br), indicates that 53% of Internet users sought information related to health or health services. This preference of Brazilians is second only to the search for information about products and services (Brazilian Network Information Center, 2022).

2.1 The "Expert Patient" and Quality of Information

Access to this health information on the Internet favors the constitution of the "expert patient": a special consumer of information about health services and products who feels somehow to have become an expert in this given subject. He is a patient who searches the Internet for information about diagnoses, diseases, symptoms, medications, hospitalization, and treatment costs. The "expert patient" would, therefore, have the potential to transform the traditional doctor-patient relationship based on the authority being concentrated in the hands of the physician (Garbin et al., 2008).

In a study we carried out on the subject, we concluded that the practice of the "expert patient" is prescribed and institutionally regulated by biomedical knowledge. For this reason, it does not seem reasonable to think that the "expert patient" is someone who, necessarily, challenges medical knowledge. However, it was possible to observe that the information consumed, produced, and shared by him contributes to his empowerment (Pereira Neto et al., 2019).

Broadly following the same argumentative framework as di Novi et al. (2024), who concluded that:

> [...] Online health information seeking behavior (e-HISB) can empower individuals to better understand health concerns, facilitating improved health condition management. (di Novi et al., 2024, p. 675)

Ryhänen et al. (2012) present the "theory of empowering knowledge" (Ryhänen et al., 2012, p. 1017). For these authors, empowerment is a cognitive state in which the individual feels greater control over his life. This dimension, despite being focused on the individual as a unit of analysis, does not consider that empowerment is a decontextualized phenomenon and one isolated from the influences arising from the relationships that subjects can establish with each other and with society.

The collective dimension of empowerment is, to a large extent, influenced by the ideas of pedagogue Paulo Freire (1987). Thus, inspired by Freire's ideas, the concept of empowerment tends to abandon the individual-psychological perspective and turn towards a necessarily collective, social, and political trend, which can present different perspectives and opinions on the same topic

This empowerment has favored shared decision-making between physician and patient about the risks and benefits of a given treatment. In this sense, Gonzalez-Argote (2022) admits that shared decision-*making* between doctor and patient: "[...] emerges as a method of patient-physician communication centered on the participation of the patient in his or her medical therapy and is credited with reducing decisional uncertainty" (Gonzalez-Argote, 2022, p. 1).

The shared decision-making process seeks to move away from the paternalistic clinical decision model. It has bioethical aspects of beneficence and non-maleficence when valuing the autonomy of the subject who is served.

In the health area, we can find virtual environments built by public and private teaching and research institutions, by government and non-governmental agencies, by patient and professional associations, and by individuals themselves. The Internet allows health information to be published and shared without any kind of evaluation, verification, or authorization. Thus, incomplete, contradictory, incorrect, or even fraudulent information may be made available. In addition, the way information is presented can be difficult to understand.

Access to low-quality health information and the sharing of it can make citizens feel empowered with misinformation. Thus, they tend to make decisions that will negatively affect their quality of life and well-being (Kuenzel et al., 2018). Incorrect, incomprehensible, or outdated information can lead citizens to make decisions harmful to their health.

Di Novi et al. (2024) reiterate the importance of providing correct information: "our findings highlight the importance of policy interventions aimed at promoting the availability of accurate and reliable health information online" (di Novi et al., 2024, p. 687).

Suarez-Lledo and Alvarez-Galvez (2021) published a systematic review whose objective was to identify the main topics of health misinformation and its prevalence on different social media platforms. The authors found 65 articles published until March 2019 in the PubMed, MEDLINE, Scopus, and Web of Science databases. They found that posts with misinformation reached 87% of the studies (Suarez-Lledo & Alvarez-Galvez, 2021).

There is also a production of purposely false health content on digital social networks. Information intended to deceive the interlocutors.

Waszak et al. (2018) concluded that:

> 40% of the most frequently shared links contained text we classified as fake news. These were shared more than 450,000 times. The most fallacious content concerned vaccines, while news about cardiovascular diseases was, in general, well sourced and informative. More than 20% of dangerous links from our material was generated by one source. (Waszak et al., 2018, p. 115)

Misinformation is bad for your health.

During the COVID-19 pandemic, the concept of *infodemic* was widespread. It combines the issue of information abundance with its rapid diffusion by offering wrong information in different formats. The Director-General of the World Health Organization, during the "Munich Safety Conference" held in 2020, declared that "We're not just fighting an epidemic; we're fighting an infodemic" (World Health Organization, 2020a).

Evaluating the quality of information is one of the ways to face the health infodemic and disinformation.

2.2 Evaluation Methods

In our view, proposals to address this challenge can be divided into three groups.

The first covers search engines like Google. When a subject is searched in them, the results are presented according to relevance criteria called *page rank*. These companies select the email addresses they consider most relevant to have on their page. The sites that usually appear at the top of the list are sponsored. In addition, the list of results of a search is generated through computational algorithms that combine various mechanisms, such as users' personal data and online search habits. These algorithms are systems capable of organizing an increasing amount of information available on the Internet. They offer daily data that can be mined, gathered, and sold. That is why, from the analysis of posts and likes on Facebook, those interested will be able to find out which politician a particular citizen is likely to vote for in the next elections or identify the probability of this person being gay. Search engines recognize the device being used by the user. These technological resources are able to gather this data and build a profile of each of us. These profiles are offered to large companies. This way, they are able to identify consumers of certain products or services. Pariser (2011) explores the problem of algorithms and their consequences, which, in his opinion, subject users to the economic interests of these companies. In *The Filter Bubble*, he demonstrates how Google, Facebook, and Amazon build search habit filters for each user based on their preferences. Such filters prevent users from accessing the full content of the web, which can be an obstacle to having a broader understanding of a subject. According to Pariser (2011), personalization is based on a bargain. In exchange for the filtering service, we offer large companies a huge amount of data about our daily lives. Information we often wouldn't share with our best friends. These companies are becoming increasingly skilled at using this data to chart their business strategies. A similar position is shared by Zhang et al. (2015). They found several studies that identified that the *page ranks* of these search engines "were not reliable predictors of a site's overall content quality" (Zhang et al., 2015, p. 2081).

The second group of initiatives proposed to address the challenge of online information quality involves collective evaluation. It concerns the evaluation systems maintained by users engaged in providing information on the quality of institutions, commercial establishments, products, services, etc. Trivago and TripAdvisor are some examples of websites that have a collective evaluation process, usually through evaluation systems performed by users of these services themselves. This model largely influences the decision-making of other consumers (Fritsch & Sigmund, 2016). Collective evaluation does not follow any standard and is guided by the evaluator's subjectivity.

The third group includes public or private institutional initiatives to assess the quality of health information on the Internet.

The main difference between the three groups lies mainly in the objectives of the evaluation and those responsible for evaluating the quality of health information on the Internet. In the first group, there is a clear business objective. Those responsible for the evaluation are private companies with their market interests. In the second, the objective is similar to that of the first group, although the users are the evaluators. In this case, the parameters used in the evaluation are too subjective, as they do not follow precise and clear quality indicators. For this reason, the outcome of these assessments may be unreliable. In the third case, the evaluation method is provided by professionals or institutions that comply with specific quality criteria.

This is, for example, the case of DISCERN.

DISCERN, created in 1998, is still one of the most utilized resources in the world for evaluating the quality of the health information on the Internet. It was created by the "Division of Public Health and Primary Health Care" of the "Institute of Health Sciences" at Oxford University (Charnock, 1998). A project managed by researchers from this division, under the coordination of Sasha Shepperd and the participation of Deborah Charnock, Gill Needham, and Robert Gann.

Charnock was the researcher responsible for editing the *DISCERN Handbook* (Charnock, 1998). It states that this assessment instrument "is suitable for anyone who uses or produces information about treatment choices" (Charnock, 1998, p. 6).

DISCERN is an assessment tool made up of 15 questions arranged in three sections. The first evaluates whether the publication is reliable, and it comprises eight questions. They guide the evaluator to verify if: the objectives of the publication are clear; the information announced is available and meets the needs of the user; there is clarity regarding the sources of information; there is a date of publication; the publication is impartial; other sources of information are offered to support the information made available; and the information encompasses the so-called gray areas where there is no certainty about how to make the diagnosis and/or provide treatment. The second section consists of five questions. They aim to guide the patient to choose the treatment they consider most convenient. They make the evaluator check if the consequences, benefits, risks, and effects of a given treatment on the patient's quality of life are found on the website. There is also a question that seeks to verify if there is any information about what can occur if that treatment is not adopted and if there are other possible treatments. The last section has only one question. It aims to guide the user to carry out an overall assessment of the quality of the publication as a source of information on treatment options. The answers are arranged in the form of a "Likert Scale" in which the evaluator answers "no," "partially," or "yes," on a range from 1 to 5. Thus, the user uses this tool to make their own evaluation of the site.

A year later, Charnock and the others responsible for building the tool published an assessment of DISCERN. They randomly assembled 15 information providers and 13 members from 19 large English self-help organizations (Charnock et al., 1999). In it, the authors concluded that:

> DISCERN is a reliable and valid instrument for judging the quality of written consumer health information. While some subjectivity is required for rating certain criteria, the findings demonstrate that the instrument can be applied by experienced users and providers of health information to discriminate between publications of high and low quality. The instrument will also be of benefit to patients, although its use will be improved by training. (Charnock et al., 1999, p. 105)

A few years later, Charnock, this time accompanied only by Shepperd, published another article (Charnock & Shepperd, 2004) to make a new evaluation of the tool they created. This time, the tool was used in the evaluation of health websites by 57 providers or consumers (patients or caregivers) of information on health websites. The authors concluded in this study that "DISCERN provides an acceptable way of appraising the quality of online consumer health information" (Charnock & Shepperd, 2004, p. 444). They warned in this text that although DISCERN was

2.2 Evaluation Methods

created to evaluate written information, "it should be applicable to online information" (Charnock & Shepperd, 2004, p. 441).

Eysenbach et al. (2002) published, 2 years before Charnock and Shepperd (2004), the first systematic review of the methods previously used to assess the quality of information on health websites. This research identified 79 articles that evaluated more than 7000 websites with 408 results that used 86 different criteria to evaluate the quality of health information available on the Internet. A criterion (from the Greek *kritérion* to the Latin *criterium*) is a standard that serves as a basis for things and people to be compared and judged. Eysenbach et al. (2002) grouped these 86 criteria into five, which were named as follows: Technical, Design, Comprehensiveness, Readability, and Accuracy. These would be the five essential attributes that information made available on health websites should have.

Let's look at how Eysenbach et al. (2002) define each of these criteria.

The "Technical" criterion is defined as that which mentions "how the information was presented or what meta-information was provided" (Eysenbach et al., 2002, p. 2694). This is the attribution of responsibility and reference for the information offered, which includes, for example, the presentation of dates of creation and updating of the website. This criterion also verifies that the website presents the authorship, attribution, dissemination, updating, and sponsorship underlying the information provided.

"Design" is concerned with the visual or aesthetic aspect of a website, such as the layout, colors, ease of navigation, the presentation of its interface, and the features available for navigation. It therefore includes the dimensions of usability and accessibility. The first checks if the site is easy to use and navigate. The second focuses on it being inclusive and allowing all people to use it, especially those with disabilities. We have come to call this criterion "Interactivity," as it refers to the ability that the user will need to have in order to deal with this device and the characteristics that it must have to facilitate this interaction.

The "Scope" verifies that the available information covers all relevant aspects of that topic or health-disease problem addressed. In the case of a contagious disease, for example, the website should provide information on transmission, prevention, symptoms, diagnosis, and treatment.

"Readability" evaluates the level of understanding of the information provided. The authors who used this criterion verified the length and complexity of the sentences and words, using formulas such as "Flesh-Kincaid" and "Grade Level Index," among others. Those are readability tests designed to indicate the difficulty of understanding a text written in English.

"Accuracy" measures the degree of agreement of information with the best medical evidence or that which is generally accepted by medical practice. Accuracy and timeliness are essential attributes for the provision of health information. Therefore, health websites need to present correct information from a scientific point of view. For Eysenbach et al. (2002), "accuracy ideally should be defined using the best available evidence" (Eysenbach et al., 2002, p. 2695). This "best evidence" would be obtained, according to the authors, in the reference works (*Textbooks*) or from the "*expert consensus.*"

Some comments seem pertinent if we compare the criteria found in the systematic review carried out by Eysenbach et al. (2002) with the 15 questions that make up the DISCERN questionnaire.

The first section of DISCERN seems to approach the concerns present in the technical criterion, especially when it asks if the sources that were used to produce that information are clear and if there is a publishing date available.

The second section of DISCERN is compromised, as it does not associate the consequences, benefits, risks, and effects of a given treatment with the current state of scientific knowledge about it.

The recent case of COVID-19 prevention can serve as an example. Many health websites in different parts of the world claimed that vaccination could cause irreparable harm and that the person receiving the vaccine would have serious health problems. Many websites presented information that, therefore, contradicts scientific knowledge. Some health websites sabotaged preventive methods such as social distancing and wearing masks. Others condemned vaccination and proposed in its place the adoption of drugs, without scientific evidence, for the prevention of COVID-19, such as Ivermectin, Chloroquine, and Hydroxychloroquine. Ivermectin is a drug used for treating diseases related to parasites. Chloroquine and Hydroxychloroquine have been used in the treatment and prophylaxis of malaria. DeJong and Wachter (2020) warned about the risks of prescribing hydroxychloroquine for the treatment of COVID-19. In Brazil, for example, these three drugs made up the so-called COVID KIT. Its adoption was supported by the Federal Government of the time. Despite this, vaccination was carried out throughout the national territory thanks to the Unified Health System (SUS). According to Furlan and Caramelli (2021), "The 'Early Treatment of Covid-19' with the 'Covid Kit' drugs is part of an international project with ongoing activities in different countries" (Furlan & Caramelli, 2021, p. 3). There were dramatic consequences to this misinformation. A survey conducted in Londrina, Paraná (Brazil), showed that 75% of Covid-19 deaths recorded in the first 10 months of 2021 occurred in individuals who were not immunized against the disease (Passarelli-Araujo et al., 2022). In Brazil, free immunization was offered by the Ministry of Health to all 5570 municipalities. People who were not immunized were certainly influenced by this information that condemned vaccination. The relation between vaccination and reduction of deaths from Covid-19 was also observed internationally (Liang et al., 2021).

Thus, a virtual environment would not be condemned if it were evaluated by the DISCERN questionnaire, if it disseminated information highlighting the possible harms of vaccination and the supposed benefits of the "COVID KIT." This site would present the benefits of treatment with Ivermectin, Chloroquine, and Hydroxychloroquine and would highlight the risks that vaccination contained. The positive consequences for the patient's quality of life with the adoption of the "COVID-KIT" would be highlighted. On this imaginary website, the information would be presented in a clear way, with explicit and recent sources, and would meet the needs of users. The website would warn the user by presenting what would occur if that treatment with the "COVID KIT" was not adopted. We want to

2.2 Evaluation Methods

highlight in this brief evaluation that the accuracy of the information is not considered in the DISCERN questionnaire.

In addition, DISCERN is not interested in verifying whether or not the user has understood what is written on the website. Readability is not part of the tool built by researchers at the University of Oxford. However, we agree with Tones (2002) when he admits that the DISCERN questionnaire could be useful to promote health literacy.

There are other initiatives to assess the quality of health information on the Internet, similar to DISCERN, among which the JAMA Benchmark and the HONcode stand out.

The "JAMA Benchmark" is a rating scale used to assess the quality and reliability of health information on the Internet. It is based on four points: *Authorship*, which verifies the attributes of the author of the information, his institutional affiliation, and other credentials. "*Attribution*," which is concerned with the references, copyright, and sources used and which serves as the basis for the information provided. *Disclosure*, referring to the website having an owner, sponsor, publicity policies, and potential conflicts of interest. *Circulation*, which identifies the date when the information was made available. The "JAMA Benchmark" was published in 1997 (Silberg et al., 1997). It is considered a simplified tool that can quickly identify websites that lack basic information transparency and reliability.

The HONcode consists of eight criteria: "Authority," which indicates the qualifications of the authors; "Complementarity," which preaches that the information should support, and not replace, the doctor-patient relationship; "Privacy," which respects the privacy and confidentiality of personal data sent to the site by the visitor; "Attribution," which reiterates the importance of citing the source(s) of published information, medical data and health pages; "Justifiability," which determines that the site should support statements related to benefits and performance; "Transparency," which values that the site should have an accessible presentation and an email for correct contact; "Funding notice," which considers the importance of the site identifying funding sources; and "Advertising Policy," which considers the importance of identify funding sources; and "Advertising Policy," which considers that a site should clearly distinguish advertising from editorial content. "Health On Net" (HON) was a certification agency that sold the HON seal of quality. HONcode was discontinued on December 15, 2022, and the website and certification review program are no longer maintained.

The HONcode and the JAMA Benchmark criteria cover only the technical dimension proposed by Eysenbach et al. (2002). These are, therefore, limited tools, as they do not consider the "accuracy" or "readability" of the information made available—two fundamental aspects for the dissemination of health information on the Internet. (Pereira Neto & Paolucci, 2019). These are two useful tools to guide the user on some care they should take when accessing a health website.

The quality and results of the systematic review carried out by Eysenbach et al. (2002), associated with the fact that it was published in the Journal of the American Medical Association, should have transformed this publication into a reference in the field of evaluation of the quality of health information on the Internet.

However, DISCERN continues to be widely used. Yang et al. (2022), for example, consider that DISCERN "is the most widely used instrument for assessing health-related information and videos, and it is particularly relevant to health-related topics and web-based resources for patient education" (Yang et al., 2022, p. 2). Baumgartner et al. (2024, p. 1) analyzed the current quality of information on jaundice found on the Internet by parents. Methodologically, "the quality of the search results was assessed by two independent neonatologists based on the DISCERN Plus Score, the HONcode certification, and the JAMA criteria" (Baumgartner et al., 2024, p. 1).

In our view, a health website should be both interactive and easily readable. In addition, the information provided must be in accordance with scientifically recognized knowledge, arranged in a technical way, and covering the different dimensions of the health problem/theme. The health information available on the website must therefore present its source, be interactive, have scientific accuracy, and be understandable by anyone.

2.3 Our Assessment Experience: Brief History

The problem of the quality of health information on the Internet has become a priority on our work agenda. In the last decade, we have carried out a set of research in the field of assessing the quality of health information on the Internet. This academic endeavor led to the publication of books, articles, book chapters, dissertations, and theses.

This academic interest led us to create, just over 10 years ago, the "Internet, Health and Society Laboratory" (LaISS) next to the Germano Sinval de Faria School Health Center, a department of the National School of Public Health (ENSP) of the Oswaldo Cruz Foundation, in Rio de Janeiro, Brazil.

This Health Center is a basic health care unit that serves a low-income and poorly educated population residing in the popular communities of Manguinhos, in the urban area of the city of Rio de Janeiro. We call this initiative a "laboratory" because we admit the possibility that this space could become an environment for experimentation and innovation. Our goal was to create an environment where Health Center users could learn to critically deal with digital technologies and help us assess the quality of information on health sites. We hoped to integrate LaISS with the other health promotion activities carried out by this ENSP department.

Our academic endeavor started from the systematic review published by Eysenbach et al. (2002) on the subject. According to these authors:

> To our knowledge, this is the first systematic review conducted to compile criteria actually used and to synthesize evaluation results from studies containing quantitative data on structure and process measures of the quality of health information on the Web. (Eysenbach et al., 2002, p. 2692).

This review found 79 distinct studies that evaluated 5941 health sites and 1329 web pages and presented 408 evaluation results for 86 different quality criteria. They were grouped by the authors into five distinct criteria that refer to specific aspects of the communication process between digital media and their users. Each of the criteria is composed of a distinct number of indicators. The indicators are directly related to the criteria. They are observable attributes associated with a website or its content, which serve as clues as to whether or not a website or its content meets a certain criterion.

As we mentioned earlier, this systematic review, published in 2002, served as a reference for our work which started in 2009. The necessary historical distance allows us to identify two moments of this methodological effort that involved the evaluation of information on health websites.

At first, we adopted the five criteria identified in the systematic review and also sought to find solutions to two problems identified by Eysenbach et al. (2002).

One of them refers to the fact that "none of the studies conducted comprehension tests with current consumers or used judgments of literacy experts" (Eysenbach et al., 2002, p. 2695). The other problem is related to the fact that the readability assessment was performed using formulas such as "Flesch-Kincaid Grade Level," among other similar formulas. The "Flesch Kincaid Grade Level" is a widely used readability formula that assesses the approximate reading level of a text, based on the average length of sentences and the complexity of English words.

Eysenbach et al. (2002) identified problems in the adoption of these readability assessment tools. They admit that:

> Using reading formulas has limitations, the readability scores do not reflect other factors that affect comprehension such as frequency and explanation of medical jargon, writing style (use of active voice, nonpatronizing language, motivational messages, tone/ mood, how it relates to the audience), or use of culturally specific information. (Eysenbach et al., 2002, p. 2694–2695)

In this first moment, we evaluated the information available on Dengue Fever, Tuberculosis, and Breastfeeding websites.

To face the first problem, we built partnerships with Fiocruz experts in their respective areas. Regarding Dengue Fever, we followed the guidance of researchers from the "Instituto Nacional de Infectologia Evandro Chagas" (Evandro Chagas National Institute of Infectious Diseases), especially colleagues from the "Laboratório de Doenças Febris Agudas" (Acute Febrile Diseases Laboratory), among which Dengue Fever stands out. In relation to tuberculosis, we counted on the collaboration of researchers from the "Professor Hélio Fraga Reference Center," dedicated to the care and research of tuberculosis. In the third case, we partnered with the specialists of the "Human Milk Bank" of the Fernandes Figueira Institute. They were the ones who defined the indicators of information accuracy for each of the health topics. That is, we used in these four cases the "expert consensus" as a resource for defining information accuracy indicators. We also invited users to build the evaluation indicators. The users, now called citizen researchers, are residents of the Communities of Manguinhos. This region is marked by inadequate housing conditions, where there is no basic sanitation, the environment is unhealthy, and cultural and leisure opportunities are practically non-existent. In addition, there is a high rate of violence and drug trafficking in the region (Fernandes & Costa, 2013). Most participants were between the ages of 30 and 40 and had not completed primary school. Thus, citizen researchers and Fiocruz researchers jointly constructed the indicators in each of the five criteria. We carried out a "Knowledge Translation": a method of research and action that aims to encourage the exchange between different types of knowledge, building a common knowledge aimed at understanding and transforming the existing reality (Barbosa & Pereira Neto, 2017).

To face the second problem, we invited the same citizen researchers and professionals who work directly in primary care at the Health Center to be the evaluators of the information, especially regarding its readability. In the experience carried out by LaISS, citizens who live in vulnerable conditions of various orders, including access to digital media, became subjects of the evaluation process by building the indicators and carrying out the evaluation.

This experience therefore brought an "incremental innovation" (Zhang, 2022, p. 2), as it improved existing processes. Zhang (2022) defines incremental innovation as follows:

> Incremental innovation is also called sustainable innovation. Incremental innovation is the gradual design of and continuous improvement in an organization's existing concepts, products, or services. It is the most common micro innovation. In incremental innovation, new technologies are rarely used. It focuses on eliminating flaws and incrementally enhancing performance through characteristics such as product line extension, cost reduction, and the next generation of products. (Zhang, 2022, p. 2).

To confirm our hypothesis, a systematic review was carried out to update the results of the effort undertaken by Eysenbach et al. (2002). This systematic review became Paolucci's master's dissertation (Paolucci, 2015), which was then published in the form of an article (Paolucci & Pereira Neto, 2021). The survey conducted in this systematic review included publications between 2001 and 2014 available in PubMed, Web of Science, LISA, LISTA, CINAHL, SciELO, BIREME, Cochrane Library, and Google Scholar databases. The protocol defined by "The Cochrane Collaboration" was followed, and is available in the *Cochrane Handbook for Systematic Reviews of Interventions* (Higgins & Green, 2008).

Some of the conclusions of this study (Paolucci & Pereira Neto, 2021) dialogue with those found in the work of Eysenbach et al. (2002) and with our concrete research experience, described and analyzed in this chapter.

One of the findings of the 2014 study was that the participation of end users in the evaluation process remained rare (Paolucci & Pereira Neto, 2021). In the studies analyzed in the systematic review carried out in 2014, the evaluators of the information available on the health websites were divided into three categories: "author" (79%), when the evaluators are the authors of the article themselves; "expert" (9%), when the evaluators are experts in the topics of the evaluated websites or invite an expert to play the role of evaluator; and "user" (5%), when the evaluators are users of the information available on the websites (Paolucci & Pereira Neto, 2021). Most of the user evaluators' category was made up of patients. Thus, the reality observed in the studies analyzed by Eysenbach et al. (2002) did not change much 12 years later.

The reality has also not changed much in relation to the procedures adopted to assess readability. The 2014 systematic review found that the two most used technologies in the studies that evaluated readability were the Flesch-Kincaid Grade Level (69%) and the Flesch Reading Ease (52%). In our case, citizen researchers were the protagonists of the evaluation process, especially regarding the dimension of information readability.

In a recent study, Peixoto et al. (2023) considered that the effort we made in this first moment to involve residents of low-income communities in the knowledge construction process is inserted in the context of "Citizen Science": a set of actions that promote the contribution of non-scientists to science, in the expectation of improving the quality of results and reducing the costs of research, in addition to expanding public engagement in science.

"Citizen science" recognizes the right to research of individuals, communities, and social groups as co-producers of knowledge. This recognition can be identified from the beginning of the investigation and at various stages of the research. This practice can contribute to new approaches and ways of doing science. It can also make the results of research processes more robust. The practice of "citizen science," therefore, provides the means and conditions for valuing the experiential knowledge of different social and cognitive actors and makes room for citizen innovation (Albagli et al., 2019).

Let us now see how the results of the evaluation of the information available on Dengue Fever, Tuberculosis, and Breastfeeding websites were obtained.

The results of the evaluation measured the degree of "compliance" between the information considered necessary, readable, and true from a scientific point of view, and the information made available on the evaluated website. The indicators were arranged in the form of interrogative sentences with two possible answers: "Yes" or "No." They indicate the presence or absence of certain information. Thus, each indicator reveals an ideal response so that the information is considered of quality. This strategy was inspired by the concept of compliance. According to the definition of the Brazilian Association of Technical Standards (ABNT), "compliance" is the "demonstration that the specified requirements [...] related to a product [...], process, system, person or body are met" (Associação Brasileira de Normas Técnicas, 2005, p. 1).

Some examples can be given in this regard. In the readability criterion, for example, there is the following question: "Did you have difficulty understanding information about Dengue Fever prevention?" This question was designed with the intention of verifying that the information provided is easy to understand. It is, therefore, an issue within the criterion of readability. It is not interested in whether the information is correct or not, nor in whether or not it has a source. The ideal—and expected—answer in this case is *no*. By checking this option, the evaluator would be informing us that, in his view, the information about transmission on that site is easy to understand. If 10 of the 20 evaluators did not have difficulty understanding the information on Dengue prevention, it means that the indicator obtained 50% compliance by the set of evaluators on that site.

In this context, ten evaluators answered that they had *no* difficulty understanding the information on Dengue prevention. Thus, in this case, we obtained only 50% of responses in accordance with what was expected and considered ideal.

The results followed the same logic in the other questions. When we add the results in each of the questions that make up this criterion, we will reach 40 answers that meet the expected out of 100 possible. As a result, this site, in the readability criterion, obtained only a 40% compliance rate.

The results of the evaluation have been consolidated into relative numbers. These percentages indicate compliance levels on each indicator within each criterion. Returning to the example mentioned above, if only ten citizen researchers, among 20 participants, find it difficult to understand the information on prevention, this site would be, according to this indicator, with 50% compliance. The average of all indicators offers the degree of compliance in that criterion of that site. The average of all criteria gives the degree of compliance of the site. Websites of government organizations such as the Ministry of Health (MS) and the State Health Departments of the Governments of Rio de Janeiro, São Paulo, and Bahia were selected. Information from non-governmental, non-profit agencies such as UNICEF was also evaluated. We also included information available on the Wikipedia website of Dr. Drauzio Varela—the most well-known science dissemination physician in Brazil, with a column on the G1 website of Globo—the biggest information and communication conglomerate in Latin America. Thus, it was possible to establish a ranking between the sites according to Tables 2.1, 2.2, and 2.3.

The number of indicators per criterion varied greatly. In this evaluation, all criteria were equally important. This view is based on the following argument: a website that offers quality health information must comply with the criteria of responsibility

Table 2.1 Evaluation of the quality of information on dengue fever websites (Pereira Neto et al., 2017)

Website/criteria	Technical	Interactivity	Scope	Accuracy	Readability	Total
Government of Rio de Janeiro	41.6	89.5	66.9	65.7	46.8	62.1
Wikipedia	61.8	44.0	71.9	38.6	53.6	52.5
Ministry of Health	37.5	76.0	57.8	62.9	28.4	52.5
Dr. Drauzio Varela	23.9	59.5	58.8	43.6	33.2	43.8
G1 Globo	26.4	48.5	35.6	22.1	30.4	32.6

Table 2.2 Evaluation of the quality of information on dengue fever websites (Paolucci et al., 2017)

Website/technical	Criterion	Interactivity	Scope	Accuracy	Readability	Total
Government of São Paulo	44	77	83	41	72	63
Ministry of Health	38	76	74	41	74	61
Wikipedia	66	59	69	38	46	56
Dr. Drauzio Varela	39	70	63	33	42	49
G1 Globo	21	70	43	29	23	37

2.3 Our Assessment Experience: Brief History

Table 2.3 Evaluation of the quality of information on breastfeeding websites (Pereira Neto et al., 2021)

Website/technical	Criterion	Interactivity	Scope	Accuracy	Readability	Total
UNICEF	47	88	77	64	64	68
Ministry of Health	43	92	56	35	38	53
Dr. Drauzio Varela	47	82	61	45	31	53
Gov. of Bahia	42	88	60	38	9	47
Wikipedia	45	62	50	42	19	44

in relation to the information provided. It must be understandable, correct, and current. It must contain information on prevention, transmission, symptoms, diagnosis, and treatment. The website, in turn, must be interactive.

The three studies performed the evaluation on a small number of websites. We admit that the number of 20 evaluators was also limited. For this reason, it becomes risky to make generalizations from these experiences. In any case, the tables reveal that most websites linked to public agencies, of public or private interest, managed to obtain a 60% compliance with the criteria and indicators used.

The results on the websites of agencies, either public or of public interest, seem worrying to us. In them, users expect to find health information scientifically updated and understandable by users of the Unified Health System.

A comment can be found on the website of the Ministry of Health.

The Ministry of Health's Dengue Fever page obtained only 28.4% in readability compliance. The Ministry of Health's breastfeeding website also proved to be incomprehensible, as it obtained a compliance rate of only 38%. These low readability rates may be associated with the fact that researchers who make information available on the website are not concerned with offering it in an understandable language. They often use scientific language instead. This was the case, for example, of the use of the word *cephalgia* to refer to one of the symptoms of Dengue Fever. The use of the word *headache* would have been easier for all users to understand.

The evaluations we did were not intended to approve or disapprove a particular digital media. Their primary function was to present a diagnosis of the situation found, revealing the aspects with greater and lesser compliance with the parameters established as ideal. Based on the diagnosis resulting from the evaluation, site managers would be able to make the indicated changes and thus increase their compliance rates.

This evaluation was the first step we took towards transforming LaISS into a certification agency for health sites. The procedure would be as follows: the site would be evaluated by a team formed by Fiocruz researchers, users of the health system, and health professionals under the coordination of LaISS, as previously described. The evaluation would reveal aspects of greater and lesser compliance present on the website. The website manager, in view of this evaluation, would make the necessary changes and resubmit the website to LaISS for further evaluation. Certainly, in this second evaluation, the compliance levels would be much higher, and the website would receive the quality seal. Thus, the user would be able to trust this certified website more than the others without certification.

The next step was to convince the board of the National School of Public Health (ENSP) of the Oswaldo Cruz Foundation of the importance of this initiative. Thus, a meeting of the Deliberative Council of the National School of Public Health was held to discuss this proposal. In December 2016, the "Internet Laboratory on Health and Society" (LaISS) had the right to grant the "Sergio Arouca Seal" to sites that met the criteria and indicators used during an evaluation. In the same year, the "Health Without Tuberculosis" Blog of the Ministry of Health received this seal. This certification initiative, however, ceased to exist. The lack of institutional support prevented this dream from coming true.

We will see below the changes we made in the methodological process of evaluating the quality of health information on the Internet.

As we noted earlier, in the three cases mentioned above (information found on Dengue Fever, Tuberculosis, and Breastfeeding websites), the indicators for evaluating the accuracy of the information were built thanks to the partnership we established with Fiocruz experts in their respective areas of knowledge and performance. Thus, we followed another conclusion presented in the systematic review carried out by Eysenbach et al. (2002) and ratified by us in a subsequent systematic review (Paolucci & Pereira Neto, 2021). In both reviews, it was found that "Textbooks or expert consensus were used as the criterion standard [...]" (Eysenbach et al., 2002, p. 2695). Thus, the accuracy of the scientific information available in the respective virtual environment was verified.

Zhang et al. (2015) also published another systematic review on the subject. They concluded that the indicators used to assess the accuracy of information continued to be defined based on the "consensus of experts," the authors themselves in their areas of expertise, and/or reference works, as had been pointed out by Eysenbach et al. (2002) and reiterated by Paolucci and Pereira Neto et al. (2021).

Zhang et al. (2015) state that:

> In 63 articles (38.2%), the instruments were created on the basis of medical guidelines, textbooks, or literature, whereas in 43 articles (26.1%), the authors, many of whom were domain experts, or invited domain experts, evaluated the content based on their medical expertise. (Zhang et al., 2015, p. 2078)

Thus, at the first moment of our investigative process, it was Fiocruz's experts who defined the information accuracy indicators that would be used for each of the health topics. That is, we used in these three cases the "expert consensus" as a resource to define the indicators of information accuracy for Dengue Fever (Pereira Neto et al., 2017), Tuberculosis (Paolucci et al., 2017), and Breastfeeding (Pereira Neto et al., 2021).

In 2020, our research carried out another "incremental innovation," as in "make new versions superior to older ones and meet more user needs" (Zhang, 2022, p. 2). This time, we abandoned the "expert consensus" and the use of reference works as a source for the creation of indicators to assess the accuracy of information. Let's see how this process unfolded.

2.3 Our Assessment Experience: Brief History

Paolucci (2020), in his doctoral thesis, criticized the construction of information accuracy indicators built from the "consensus of experts." In an article published as a result of this Thesis, we state that the "expert consensus":

> [...] does not guarantee that the result of this consensus is current and correct. On the contrary, the professionals involved may be outdated in relation to the best scientific evidence. They can also present opinions and conduct that might be in disuse (Paolucci et al., 2021, p. 140).

Corroborating this view, Betting et al. (2003) state that the "expert consensus" is achieved through the participants' answers to specific clinical questions. Responses are summarized and organized to construct guidelines that can be deployed, for example, in practical documents of medical recommendations and in care and institutional protocols. Generally, few people participate in this consensus.

Nadanovsky (1999), when evaluating the limitations of the "expert consensus," states that there is an "inability of the physician to keep up with important steps forward" (Nadanovsky, 1999, p. 22). For him, "extraordinary variations in the physician's clinical behavior and in the rates of beneficial, useless and harmful interventions" are observable (Nadanovsky, 1999, p. 22).

It is worth remembering that the definition of Eysenbach et al. (2002) of the criterion of accuracy of scientific information in the evaluation process relates to the idea that it should measure the "degree of concordance of the information provided with the best evidence or with generally accepted medical practice" (Eysenbach et al., 2002, p. 2695). The degree of agreement of information with medical practice is usually achieved through the consensus of a small number of specialists. For Nadanovsky (1999), this process does not necessarily guarantee that the result is current and correct. On the contrary, the professionals involved may be outdated in relation to the best scientific evidence. They may also display opinions and conduct that are in disuse.

Thus, in our view, the construction of indicators to assess the scientific accuracy of the information available on health websites should no longer be carried out through "expert consensus" or reference works.

Our effort, in this second moment, was to discover a way to build indicators to assess the scientific accuracy of health information on the Internet that would not be guided by the "expert consensus." This is how we approached the concept of "evidence-based medicine" (EBM). This became the resource for the construction of accuracy indicators in the evaluation of health information available on the Internet.

Let's look initially at what this expression means: "evidence-based medicine" (EBM). According to Sackett et al. (1996):

> Evidence based medicine is the conscientious, explicit, and judicious use of current best evidence in making decisions about the care of individual patients. The practice of evidence based medicine means integrating individual clinical expertise with the best available external clinical evidence from systematic research. (Sackett et al., 1996, p. 71)

Alper and Haynes (2016) created a model to obtain the best evidence after more than 15 years of research. These authors built an illustrated model through a pyramid consisting of five levels, using the letter S five times: Studies, Systematic Reviews, Systematically Derived Recommendations, Synthesized Summaries for Clinical Reference, and Systems, organized in the form of a pyramid.

At the base of the pyramid are the "original studies" that analyze specific cases of some disease or health event. In the second are the "systematic reviews" that bring together hundreds of articles that address the same disease or health event. At the third level are syntheses or "guidelines": statements designed to help end users, managers, and health professionals make informed decisions about whether, when, and how to perform specific actions, such as clinical, surgical interventions, diagnostic tests, or public health measures, with the aim of achieving the best possible individual or collective health outcomes. The fourth level presents a "synthesized summary for clinical reference" based on evidence from the three previous levels, namely: original study, systematic review, and *guideline*. For Alper and Haynes (2016, p. 124):

> Synthesised summaries for clinical reference provide frequently updated summaries of evidence and systematically derived recommendations and become the top level when searching for practical guidance for EBHC. Current resources providing synthesised summaries for clinical reference with varying degrees of quality, currency and comprehensiveness include BMJ Best Practice, DynaMed Plus, EBM Guidelines, Essential Evidence Plus and UpToDate.

Dicenso et al. (2009) reveal that, until recently, to obtain the best evidence, we needed to learn techniques to search the specialized literature and develop critical assessment skills to identify and understand quality clinical studies. Bibliographic search tools, bibliographic databases, and systematic reviews and other resources are possible thanks to the use of digital media. They made it easier to get the best evidence quickly and accurately. According to them:

> The application of high-quality evidence to clinical decision making requires that we know how to access that evidence. In years past, this literature meant searching know-how and application of critical appraisal skills to separate lower from higher quality clinical studies. However, over the past decade, many practical resources have been created to facilitate ready access to high-quality research. (Dicenso et al., 2009, p. 99)

There are currently "many practical resources" (Dicenso et al., 2009, p. 99) that offer on the Internet "synthesized summaries" with medical information based on evidence.

Alper and Haynes (2016) had mentioned that *BMJ Best Practice*, *DynaMed Plus*, *EBM Guidelines*, *Essential Evidence Plus,* and UpToDate were sources that offered "synthesised summaries for clinical reference." Kwag et al. (2016) reported that, in recent years, the number of organizations offering this service has increased. They conducted an evaluation study of these initiatives and concluded that *Best Practice,*[1] *DynaMed,*[2] *and UptoDate scored highest on all dimensions, whereas other*

---

[1] Available at: https://bestpractice.bmj.com/

[2] Available at: https://www.dynamed.com/

2.3 Our Assessment Experience: Brief History

companies, which market the same service, have less reliable evidence.[3] In this study, Kwag et al. (2016) concluded that:

> Medical and scientific publishers are investing substantial resources towards the development and maintenance of point-of-care summaries. The number of these products has increased since 2008 along with their quality. Best Practice, Dynamed, and UptoDate scored the highest across all dimensions, while others that were marketed as evidence-based were less reliable. Individuals and institutions should regularly assess the value of point-of-care summaries as their quality changes rapidly over time. (Kwag et al., 2016, p. 1)

Bradley-Ridout et al. (2021) conducted a study with the objective "to compare the accuracy, time to answer, user confidence, and user satisfaction between *UpToDate* and *DynaMed* (formerly DynaMed Plus), which are two popular point-of-care information tools" (Bradley-Ridout et al., 2021, p. 382).

They concluded that "despite a preference for *UpToDate* and a higher confidence in responses, the accuracy of clinical answers in *UpToDate* was equal to those in *DynaMed*. Previous exposure to *UpToDate* likely played a major role in participants' preferences" (Bradley-Ridout et al., 2021, p. 382).

DynaMed presents itself as a dynamic initiative.

> DynaMed's living topics are regularly updated as new evidence is identified through the systematic literature surveillance process. In addition, topics undergo updating and review by the editorial team. This process includes performing subject area-specific targeted queries across the over 5,000 journals indexed in PubMed. This ensures that DynaMed includes the most current evidence for use at the point of care. (EBSCO Information Services, 2024)

DynaMed therefore offers up-to-date, quality, evidence-based information that is easily located in a database. Access to the platform is not free: to consult the available content, the interested party must pay an annual subscription, the amount of which varies according to the user's profile.

In this second moment, we started to use *DynaMed* as a resource for the construction of indicators of accuracy of scientific information in the evaluation of the quality of health information available on the Internet. Thus, we abandoned the perspective of obtaining the accuracy of scientific information through the "expert consensus."

Building indicators of the accuracy of scientific information using "synthesised summaries for clinical reference" is something innovative. We are not aware of a single study that has used this resource. An analysis was carried out to identify these initiatives in Brazil (Barbosa et al., 2023). This study from 2021 carried out the research in the main Brazilian bibliographic databases. At the time, 30 articles and 18 dissertations and theses on assessing the quality of health information on the Internet were identified.

Its authors concluded that:

> Regarding the way the analyzed publications evaluate the accuracy of the information, three main resources were identified: consensus between authors and/or experts; manuals, *guidelines* and/or books; and bibliographic studies and/or systematic reviews. [...] None of the

---

[3] Available at: https://www.uptodate.com/

analyzed publications used scientific evidence systems or synthesized summaries for clinical references—considered the best levels of scientific evidence available. (Barbosa et al., 2023, p. 278)

We performed two assessments of the accuracy of scientific health information available on the Internet, using the *DynaMed* tool. One became Paolucci's Thesis (2020), recently published in article format. She analyzed the quality of tuberculosis information (Paolucci et al., 2022). The other one was the result of research carried out at the Fiocruz unit of the Mato Grosso do Sul state when the quality of leishmaniasis information was analyzed (Pereira Neto et al., 2023). In both cases, the information was provided in links on the "Health from A to Z" Portal of the Ministry of Health.

This Portal is a glossary that makes available health information. It is hosted on the website of the Ministry of Health. The information it provides can therefore be considered reliable. It is an information reference for citizens and managers. Indicators were created to evaluate the accuracy of information for tuberculosis and leishmaniasis in order to compare the existing information from the Ministry of Health Portal with that found in *DynaMed* for each of these diseases.

Let's look at leishmaniasis first.

In relation to the evaluation of information on leishmaniasis, 20 indicators were constructed, 6 of which relate to transmission, 4 to symptoms and diagnosis, 7 to prevention, and 4 to treatment (Pereira Neto et al., 2023).

Results were surprising: Of the six relevant pieces of information on leishmaniasis transmission, only three were complete. None of the five symptoms information on the *DynaMed* website was available in the Ministry of Health glossary. In prevention, only three of the seven information recommended by *DynaMed* were available on the Portal. What caught our attention was the fact that no information about treatment was available on the "Health from A to Z" Portal (Pereira Neto et al., 2023).

Another aspect that deserves to be highlighted is the absence of certain important information. The Portal states that:

> Visceral Leishmaniasis is transmitted through the bite of insects popularly known as "mosquito palha" (straw mosquito), asa dura (hardwing), tatuquira, birigui, among others. These insects are small and have yellowish or straw-colored characteristics and, in a resting position, their wings remain erect and semi-open. (Ministry of Health, 2023)

It is stated in DynaMed that "Female phlebotomine sandflies only vector for transmission. Noiseless, 2–3 mm long arthropods (about one-third the size of mosquitoes)." This information was obtained by *DynaMed* in some scientific articles highlighting the guidance of the "Centers for Disease Control and Prevention" (CDC) for leishmaniasis published in 2013.

In the Portal of the Ministry of Health, it did not inform, therefore, the size of the insect or the fact that it is silent. We ask: How can someone identify the insect transmitting the disease if the website of the Ministry of Health of Brazil does not provide this information?

In the same article, we evaluated the accuracy of information on pages about leishmaniasis on the websites of "Médecins Sans Frontières/Doctors Without Borders" (MSF) and the "Drugs for Neglected Diseases Initiative" (DNDi). These are internationally recognized non-governmental organizations that develop safe, effective, and affordable treatments for millions of vulnerable people who are affected by neglected diseases. We also assessed the quality of information on leishmaniasis on the government website of India: one of the countries most affected by this disease worldwide. These three websites have, therefore, broad notorious public recognition and, due to their institutional linkage, can be perceived as credible sources of health information.

The results of this investigation are equally surprising. None of the three websites reports that the transmitting insect is most active from dusk to dawn, although some species are active during the day. For this reason, they also do not inform that one of the ways to prevent contagion is to avoid outdoor activities, especially from dusk to dawn. In addition, *DynaMed* recommends that outdoors, in endemic areas, people wear trousers and long-sleeved shirts. On the DNDi website, it is recommended that patients with visceral leishmaniasis undergo "an oral, effective, safe, low-cost, and short-term treatment," without making any mention of the most commonly adopted type of drug.

Citizens who live in endemic areas and consult one of the *websites* of the two NGOs will not find the necessary information to prevent and take proper care of themselves, as there is no information on how to behave in this epidemiological context.

DynaMed contains the following information:

> Treatment should be guided by expert consultation. Treatment decision may vary by infecting species, geographic location, local resistance pattern, patient characteristics, availability of medications. For treatment of visceral leishmaniasis, all patients should be treated [...]. Liposomal amphotericin B is generally considered the first line due to a higher cure rate and lower side effect profile when compared to older agents. (DynaMed, 2022)

DynaMed based its information on a publication in the "Clinical Practice Guidelines by the Infectious Diseases Society of America (IDSA) and the American Society of Tropical Medicine and Hygiene" (Aronson et al., 2016).

The table below gathers the final results of the research in which we evaluated the quality of information about leishmaniasis on important public and public-interest websites.

The first column refers to each of the evaluation criteria. The second presents the total points possible if the information were 100% in compliance with the indicators created from *DynaMed (Gold Standard)*. The following columns show the results obtained by each site evaluated in each of the four criteria, revealing the highest or lowest degree of compliance with the expected result. In the end, the results were transformed into proportional indicators (Table 2.4).

As noted above, the information available on visceral leishmaniasis in four important virtual environments was given low rates of compliance with the current scientific knowledge presented in the summary synthesized for clinical reference,

Table 2.4 Results of the accuracy of information on visceral leishmaniasis (Pereira Neto et al., 2023)

Criterion	Total	MSF	DNDi	MS/B	MS/I
Transmission	60	5	5	35	20
Symptoms and diagnosis	40	10	5	10	15
Prevention	70	0	0	35	50
Treatment	30	5	0	0	15
Total	200	20	10	80	100
Percentage		10%	5%	40%	50%

MSF—Doctors without orders, DNDi—"Drugs for Neglected Diseases Initiative", MS/B—Ministry of Health. Brazil, MS/I—Ministry of Health. India

provided in *DynaMed*. Most of the information provided, in this case, is incomplete, incorrect, or missing despite the fact that the websites are linked to reputable institutions. It cannot be said that this disinformation was deliberately intended to deceive. However, it is important to note that some important information available on these sites is not correct or is missing.

In relation to tuberculosis, 43 indicators of information accuracy were constructed and proposed. Thirty-one of them were not present in the link dedicated to tuberculosis in the "Health from A to Z" Portal. Thus, most of the information on tuberculosis, based on evidence-based medicine, is absent from the glossary analyzed. There is also information that has been found to be wrong. This is the aspect we have highlighted in this chapter. It may surprise many of us, but we are facing a public website linked to the Brazilian Ministry of Health that provides outdated information or does not provide all the most relevant information about tuberculosis: the second leading cause of death by a single infectious agent in Brazil, surpassed only by the coronavirus disease SARS-CoV-2 (Ministry of Health, 2024).

Much of the information on tuberculosis available on *DynaMed* follows the guidelines of the third edition of the "International Standards for Tuberculosis Care" (ISTC), published in 2014 (TB CARE I, 2014). The purpose of ISTC is to:

> [...] to provide support to the integrated, patient-centered care and prevention component of WHO's global strategy for tuberculosis prevention, care, and control after 2015. Engagement of all providers is a critical component of the updated strategy and the ISTC will serve as a means of facilitating implementation of the strategy, especially among private providers. (TB CARE I, 2014, p. 6)

It is stated in the ISTC document that:

> all patients, including children, with unexplained cough lasting *two or more weeks* [emphasis added] or with unexplained findings suggestive of tuberculosis on chest radiographs should be evaluated for tuberculosis.
> [...] The most commonly reported symptom of pulmonary tuberculosis is persistent cough that generally, but not always, is productive of mucus and *sometimes blood (hemoptysis)* [emphasis added]. In persons with tuberculosis the cough is often accompanied by systemic symptoms such as fever, night sweats, and weight loss. (TB CARE I, 2014, p. 21)

Let's stick, at this point, to these two symptoms suggestive of tuberculosis: the period of coughing and hemoptysis.

2.3 Our Assessment Experience: Brief History

The Glossary page "Health from A to Z" dedicated to tuberculosis states that the symptoms of this disease are "Cough for *three weeks* [emphasis added] or more, afternoon fever, night sweats and weight loss" (Ministry of Health, 2022). At the end, there is a sentence that indicates that "the main symptom of pulmonary tuberculosis is cough. This cough can be dry or productive (with phlegm)" (Ministry of Health, 2022). There is a sentence, highlighted with the following content:

> *Important* [author's emphasis]: It is recommended that anyone with respiratory symptoms, that is, who has a *cough for three weeks* or more [emphasis added], be investigated for tuberculosis. (Ministry of Health, 2022)

As we can see, the link dedicated to tuberculosis on the Ministry of Health Portal does not inform that hemoptysis is a symptom of tuberculosis; this information is missing! Another problem is the presence in the glossary of outdated information about the duration of the cough as a symptom suggestive of tuberculosis.

We were surprised by this outdatedness, especially because the information on hemoptysis and the 2 weeks of coughing was already present in the previous edition of the ISTC, published in 2009. The version published in 2014 contains a table with the "key differences between the 2009 and 2014 editions of the ISTC" (TB CARE I, 2014, p. 6). In this update, there is no information that contradicts the 2-week duration of symptoms suggestive of tuberculosis or the fact that sputum is often accompanied by blood.

Thus, the duration of coughing as a symptom suggestive of tuberculosis in the ISTC is shorter than the time reported in the glossary of the Ministry of Health. Compliance with the 2-week cough period for the early diagnosis of tuberculosis can contribute to the beginning of treatment, increasing the possibility of cure and decreasing the ability to transmit the disease, as the infected patient could take steps not to transmit tuberculosis to their families and neighbors. This information oriented the procedures in the health services. It became a care protocol. The fact that the health professional waits 3 weeks to start the diagnostic tests and does not consider hemoptysis as a symptom of the disease can have serious consequences! It can facilitate the transmission of the disease, reduce patient resistance, and anticipate death. Outdated information can harm the patient!

This is only one of the many examples that could be given about the benefits that quality information can provide to the life of the citizen. This is only one of the many examples serving as evidence that outdated, wrong, or incomprehensible information may favor the transmission of a disease, inhibit preventive measures, increase cure practices uncertified by science, and, more extremely, anticipate death.

Brazil is not the only country to offer health information in an *online* glossary.

The "National Health Service" of the United Kingdom has a website that hosts a glossary, similar to the Brazilian one, called "Health A to Z" (National Health Service, 2019). It offers information on different situations and conditions of health and disease. About the symptoms of tuberculosis, the following information is available:

> Symptoms of tuberculosis (TB) usually come on gradually. Common symptoms include: a cough that lasts *more than 3 weeks*—you may cough up mucus (phlegm) or mucus with

blood in it; feeling tired or exhausted; a high temperature or night sweats; loss of appetite; weight loss and feeling generally unwell. (National Health Service, 2023)

The US government also has a similar initiative. The "National Institutes of Health" (NIH) provides a link, in Spanish, dedicated to offering health information called "MedlinePlus Informacíon de salud para usted" ("MedlinePlus: Health Information for You") (MedlinePlus, 2019a). It also has a glossary. It offers information on different situations and conditions of health and disease. This virtual environment, originally published in Spanish, contains the following information about the symptoms of tuberculosis:

> With tuberculosis, symptoms will depend on where tuberculosis is growing in your body. General symptoms may include: Chills and fever; Night sweats (heavy sweating during sleep); Weight loss; Loss of appetite; Weakness or fatigue. Symptoms of tuberculosis in the lungs may include; cough lasting *more than three weeks* [emphasis added]; coughing up blood or sputum (thick mucus from the lungs); chest pain. (MedlinePlus, 2019b)

The Government of Catalonia in Spain also maintains a website where it provides information on different situations and conditions of health and illness (Generalitat de Catalunya, 2024a). It also has a link called "Salut A–Z," originally published in Catalan. "Símptomes de la tuberculosi" ("Symptoms of Tuberculosis") states that:

> The symptoms and signs of tuberculosis vary according to the affected organ. In the case of pulmonary tuberculosis, which is the most frequent and contagious form, the most common symptom is persistent cough; that is, one that lasts *more than three weeks* [emphasis added]. (Generalitat de Catalunya, 2024b)

The Government of the State of Quebec in Canada also maintains a website with health information in French called "Problèmes de Santé de A à Z" (Health Problems from A to Z) (Gouvernement du Québec, 2025). It also contains a link dedicated to tuberculosis. With regard to its symptoms, the following information appears:

> Symptoms of active TB depend on which part of the body is infected. When tuberculosis lodges in the lungs (pulmonary tuberculosis), its main symptoms are: *cough that lasts more than 3 weeks* [emphasis added], often accompanied by sputum; fever; great tiredness; loss of appetite; night sweats; weight loss. (Gouvernement du Québec, 2024)

The information on the symptoms suggestive of tuberculosis is therefore outdated on the official websites of public institutions that we analyze in this chapter. This false information may have an explanation.

The "International Standards for Tuberculosis Care," published in January 2006 by the "Tuberculosis Coalition for Technical Assistance (TB-CTA)" states the following "Standard 1" for the Diagnosis of Tuberculosis:

> The most common symptom of pulmonary tuberculosis is persistent, productive cough, often accompanied by systemic symptoms, such as fever, night sweats, and weight loss.
> [...] Although the presence of *cough for 2–3 weeks* [emphasis added] is nonspecific, traditionally, having cough of this duration has served as the criterion for defining suspected tuberculosis and is used in most national and international guidelines, particularly in areas of moderate-to high prevalence of tuberculosis. (TB-CTA, 2006, p. 17)

Thus, we can assume that the official portals of different national or regional governments, mentioned above, have offered the information set out in the 2006 document. It contains the cough of 2–3 weeks and does not include hemoptysis as symptoms suggestive of pulmonary tuberculosis. That is a mere assumption. It seems surprising to us if we take into account that the accepted international standards were released in 2014: 10 years ago!

The presentation of the third edition of the "International Standards for Tuberculosis Care" (ISTC), published in 2014 (TB CARE I, 2014) contains a brief description of its construction process.

> Edition 3 was again funded by USAID via TB CARE I and was developed using essentially the same process. Development was led by Mukund Uplekar (WHO) and Philip Hopewell (ATS). [...] The standards in the ISTC are all supported by existing WHO guidelines and policy statements, many of which have recently been developed using rigorous methodology, including systematic reviews. The draft document was then reviewed by an expert committee of 27 members from 13 countries, co-chaired by Drs. Uplekar and Hopewell. Subsequent drafts were also reviewed and approved by the expert committee. The final draft was reviewed and approved by the TB CARE I member organizations (ATS, FHI 360, the Japan Antituberculosis Association [JATA], KNCV Tuberculosis Foundation [KNCV], Management Sciences for Health [MSH], the International Union against Tuberculosis and Lung Disease [The Union], and WHO). (TB CARE I, 2014, p. 4)

2.4 Final Considerations

We are not experts in tuberculosis. We based this reflection on the official documents of important scientific institutions of international renown in order to structure our argument.

The misinformation present in the virtual environments mentioned above can have serious consequences.

In March 2025, the World Health Organization reported that:

> A total of 1.25 million people died from tuberculosis (TB) in 2023 (including 161 000 people with HIV). Worldwide, TB has probably returned to being the world's leading cause of death from a single infectious agent, following three years in which it was replaced by coronavirus disease (COVID-19). It was also the leading killer of people with HIV and a major cause of deaths related to antimicrobial resistance.
>
> [...] Ending the TB epidemic by 2030 is among the health targets of the United Nations Sustainable Development Goals (SDGs). (World Health Organization, 2025)

In our view, quality information, updated and scientifically based, can assist in the fulfillment of this goal. Outdated information, such as that presented above, can pose a serious obstacle in this regard.

Should providing quality information to the population be an obligation of institutions, either public or of public interest? Is this a way to combat unhealthy misinformation?

The proposal I present in this chapter is part of a current international debate.

Eysenbach (2020) published an article during the COVID-19 pandemic that became an important reference. In it, the author recovered the expressions that he himself had created as in "infodemic" (Eysenbach, 2020, p. 1), "infodemiology" (Eysenbach, 2002, p. 763; Eysenbach, 2006, p. 244), "infoveillance" (Eysenbach, 2009, p. 1). "Infodemiology" is defined as a new emerging discipline that includes the study of determinants and the distribution of health disinformation.

> It is not without pride that I witnessed how this line of research is now formally acknowledged by public health organizations and the WHO as a novel, emerging scientific field and critical area of practice during a pandemic. (Eysenbach, 2020, p. 1)

The article by Eysenbach (2020) was published at the beginning of the pandemic. In that context, the dispute between scientific truths was evident in the international scenario. On the occasion, Eysenbach (2020) stated:

> [...] however, what we have learned in 20 years of infodemiology research is that the quality of health information is *an elusive concept* [emphasis added], as in medicine, the truth is not always easy to determine, especially in a rapidly evolving situation. (Eysenbach, 2020, p. 1)

For us, health information is not an "elusive concept" (Eysenbach, 2020, p. 1). The "summaries synthesized for clinical reference" presented in this chapter represent the basis for identifying scientific truth and can be useful for building indicators of scientific accuracy of the information available in virtual environments. Despite being provisional, as science is constantly under construction, it is possible to obtain quality information.

In the same article, Eysenbach (2020) modifies his argument by stating:

> While certain technical quality criteria, readability scores, and compliance with ethical quality criteria (such as the presence of disclosure of who owns the site and conflicts of interests, all aspects that are important to determine the source credibility) are relatively easy to measure, the concepts of *accuracy, facts,* and *truth* [author's emphasis] *usually require the presence of evidence-based guidelines or systematic reviews* [emphasis added] as a gold standard to determine what works and what does not. (Eysenbach, 2020, p. 2)

This was exactly the effort we undertook in this chapter and in the last 15 years of research: building a method of evaluating the accuracy of information that escapes the consensus of experts and the commonly used reference books. The information obtained in "summaries synthesized for clinical reference" can become a "gold standard" to attest to the presence or absence of certain current and scientifically based information. The "gold standard" of health information is available on sites such as *Best Practice, DynaMed,* and *UptoDate,* reviewed in this chapter.

Eysenbach (2020) presents in the same article four "pillars" for the confrontation of false information.

The first pillar of coping suggested by the author aims to make knowledge understandable to different audiences. He emphasizes that *"The first pillar of infodemic management is to support, facilitate, and strengthen accurate knowledge translation"* [author's emphasis] (Eysenbach, 2020, p. 3).

> [...] these knowledge translation processes are, perhaps, the *main mechanisms* [emphasis added] where information becomes misinformation, as the interpretation of 'facts' is sub-

2.4 Final Considerations

ject to multiple potentially influencing factors such as politics, commercial interests, selective reporting, and misunderstandings. (Eysenbach, 2020, p. 3)

The second pillar aims to refine and filter knowledge and verify facts. For Eysenbach (2020):

> on the science level, the process of *peer reviewing* [emphasis added] and publishing scholarly work is a method to constantly filter, refine, and improve the information generated by previous scholars. (Eysenbach, 2020, p. 4)

This is one of the criticisms we set out in this chapter. For us, *peer review* is not able to filter, refine, and improve the information offered by health portals. "Summaries synthesized for clinical reference" perform this function more fully and accurately.

The third pillar is focused on the construction of "eHealth literacy," defined as "the ability to seek, find, understand, and appraise health information from electronic sources and apply the knowledge gained to addressing or solving a health problem." According to the author:

> In the information age (which is now perhaps shifting to the infodemic age!) the user carries a significant part of the responsibility to select and downstream-filter trustworthy health information. [...] Thus, *the third pillar of infodemic management is to enhance the capacity of all stakeholders to build eHealth literacy, to select and assess health and science information found on the different layers of the information cake* [author's emphasis]. This aspect is notably underdeveloped in the WHO paper's taxonomy but can be seen as part of WHO's "identify evidence" category. (Eysenbach, 2020, p. 4)

This will be the theme of the next chapter.

The fourth pillar refers to "infodemic management," defined by him as the "continuous monitoring and analysis of data and information exchange patterns on the Internet."

In these terms, it compares epidemiological surveillance with infodemiological surveillance.

> My idea was that similar to surveillance in pandemics we want to be able to detect outbreaks of misinformation, rumors, falsehoods, to counter them with facts or other interventions. *Infoveillance* [emphasis added] requires generating metrics on information supply on the internet, including its quality [...], as well as information demand metrics, such as search queries or questions posed on social media or other web 2.0 platforms. (Eysenbach, 2020, p. 4)

This fourth pillar refers to a public policy of infoveillance.

In the same year, a group of researchers from the World Health Organization (WHO) published an article in which they identified more than 500 ideas and actions to manage the "infodemic," defined as:

> [...] an overabundance of information—some accurate and some not—that occurs during an epidemic. In a similar manner to an epidemic, it spreads between humans via digital and physical information systems. (Tangcharoensathien et al., 2020, p. 2)

These initiatives were grouped into 50 actions. They revealed six implications. First, interventions and messages should be based on science and evidence, and should reach citizens and empower them to make informed decisions about how to protect themselves. Knowledge must be understood and accessible by all individuals in all parts of all societies. It should promote behavior change. Third, governments must engage with communities to ensure that their concerns and information needs are understood. Fourth, to facilitate the impact of information, strategic partnerships must be established with all sectors, including academia and civil society. Fifth, health authorities must ensure that their actions are based on reliable information. Finally, infodemic management approaches should guide the user in risk mitigation.

We note that there is, both in the World Health Organization (WHO) document (Tangcharoensathien et al., 2020) and in the text of Eysenbach (2020), a concern to make information understandable by everyone.

This concern was present in the first moment of our methodological process of evaluating the quality of information. At that time, users of the public health system identified degrees of greater or lesser understanding of the information available in different virtual health environments. They were "citizen scientists."

In the second moment, we limit ourselves to building a method of measuring the (always provisional) truth of medical science. We are not concerned with the translation of knowledge. Our intention was not to verify how much the available information would be understandable by this or that social group. This may have been the shortcoming of the proposal presented in this chapter.

In future studies, we intend to associate the evaluation of the quality of health information, based on evidence-based medicine, with the transformation of the available text to "Plain Language."

Stoll M et al. (2022) understand that:

> Good research practices include publication and dissemination of results as well as their honest and transparent communication. It is further argued that the public, or at least relevant stakeholders, should have access to research, not only technically but also intellectually. This means that the public needs to be able to understand what the researchers have done, what the results mean and which practical implications can be drawn from them. […] The traditional communication of scientific findings therefore constitutes a scientific 'bubble' in which scientists communicate with each other about the meaning of their findings. As is typical for such group formation processes, this bubble results in its own special type of language, shared knowledge as well as implicit and explicit norms, which makes scientific communication harder to understand for those outside the scientific bubble. Such a context provides a breeding ground for the evolution of idiosyncratic professional jargon. This lack of plain, easily comprehensible language hinders the public from directly accessing scientific articles. (Stoll M et al., 2022, p. 1–2)

Thus, "Simple Language" is a form of communication used to convey scientific information in a simple, objective, and inclusive way. In addition to being a technique, it is also a social cause, as it defends the effective access of citizens to public services and the full understanding of their rights and duties (Cappelli et al., 2023). "Simple Language" is a broad concept that refers to different approaches and initiatives aimed at simplifying written and oral language, making it more accessible and understandable to a broad audience, including people with low literacy or cognitive disabilities. These initiatives aim to reduce complexity and the use of jargon, thus facilitating communication and ensuring that information is accessible to all.

If public and public-interest websites act in this way, they will be following one of the guidelines of the World Health Organization at its 73rd World Assembly to combat the COVID-19 pandemic, namely:

> to provide the population with reliable and comprehensive information on COVID-19 and the measures taken by authorities in response to the pandemic, and to take measures to counter misinformation and disinformation as well as malicious cyber activities. (World Health Organization, 2020b)

The WHO called on international organizations and other relevant stakeholders to:

> Address, and where relevant in coordination with Member States, the proliferation of disinformation and misinformation particularly in the digital sphere, as well as the proliferation of malicious cyber-activities that undermine the public health response, and support the timely provision of clear, objective and science-based data and information to the public. (World Health Organization, 2020b)

The main question is how to "provide the population with reliable and comprehensive information" or how to "support the timely provision of clear, objective and science-based data and information to the public."

This chapter sought to present an innovative method of evaluating the accuracy of information made available on health websites. Innovation is associated with the method we propose: not to carry out the evaluation following the point of view of experts or manuals, but from evidence-based medicine. Following this strategy, public and public-interest virtual environments from different countries and regions were evaluated. Some important information they present is outdated. Others are absent.

We emphasize that the evaluation method proposed here can be adapted to verify the informative content on other diseases and health conditions. It can bring important results about the accuracy of scientific information circulating online on other health topics. The next step to be taken is related to the translation of knowledge. Often, public or public-interest websites offer accurate and up-to-date information in incomprehensible ways.

References

Albagli, S., Parra, H., Fonseca, F. S., et al. (2019). Open science and social change: A case study in Brazil. In L. Chan, L. Okune, R. Hillyer, et al. (Eds.), *Contextualizing openness: Situating open science* (pp. 291–310). University of Ottawa Press.

Alper, B. S., & Haynes, R. B. (2016). EBHC pyramid 5.0 for accessing preappraised evidence and guidance. *Evidence-Based Medicine, 21*(4), 123–125.

Aronson, N., Herwaldt, B. L., Libman, M., et al. (2016). Diagnosis and treatment of Leishmaniasis: Clinical practice guidelines by the Infectious Diseases Society of America (IDSA) and the American Society of Tropical Medicine and Hygiene (ASTMH). *Clinical Infectious Diseases, 63*(12), 1539–1557.

Associação Brasileira de Normas Técnicas. (2005). *Avaliação de conformidade - Vocabulário e princípios gerais. ABNT NBR ISO/IEC 17000*. ABNT.

Barbosa, L., & Pereira Neto, A. (2017). Ludwik Fleck (1896-1961) e a translação do conhecimento: considerações sobre a genealogia de um conceito. *Saúde Debate, 41*, 317–329.

Barbosa, L., Pereira Neto, A., & Felipette, J. (2023). Avaliação da qualidade da informação de saúde on-line: uma análise bibliográfica da produção acadêmica brasileira [Evaluation of the quality of online health information: A bibliographic analysis of Brazilian academic production]. *Saúde debate, 47*(137), 272–283.

Baumgartner, M. K., Behr, A. L., Garbe, A. C., et al. (2024). Diving into the digital landscape: Assessing the quality of online information on neonatal jaundice for parents. *Children, 11*(7), 877.

Betting, L. E., Kobayashi, E., Montenegro, M. A., et al. (2003). Tratamento de epilepsia: consenso dos especialistas brasileiros [Treatment of epilepsy: Consensus of the Brazilian specialists]. *Arquivos de Neuro-Psiquiatria, 61*(4), 1045–1070.

Bradley-Ridout, G., Nekolaichuk, E., Jamieson, T., et al. (2021). UpToDate versus DynaMed: A cross-sectional study comparing the speed and accuracy of two point-of-care information tools. *Journal of the Medical Library Association, 109*(3), 382–387.

Brazilian Network Information Center – NIC.br. (2022). *Survey on the use of information and communication technologies in Brazilian households: ICT Households 2021*. Comitê Gestor da Internet no Brasil.

Capelli, C., Oliveira, R., & Nunes, V. (2023). Linguagem simples como pilar da transparência. *Humanidades & Inovação, 10*(9), 32–45.

Charnock, D. (1998). *The DISCERN Handbook. Quality criteria for consumer health information on treatment choices*. Radcliffe Medical Press.

Charnock, D., & Shepperd, S. (2004). Learning to DISCERN online: Applying an appraisal tool to health websites in a workshop setting. *Health Education Research, 19*(4), 440–446.

Charnock, D., Shepperd, S., Needham, G., et al. (1999). DISCERN: An instrument for judging the quality of written consumer health information on treatment choices. *Journal of Epidemiology and Community Health, 53*(2), 105–111.

DeJong, C., & Wachter, R. M. (2020). The risks of prescribing hydroxychloroquine for treatment of COVID-19 –First, do no harm. *JAMA Internal Medicine, 180*(8), 1118–1119.

di Novi, C., Kovacic, M., & Orso, C. E. (2024). Online health information seeking behavior, healthcare access, and health status during exceptional times. *Journal of Economic Behavior and Organization, 220*, 675–690.

Dicenso, A., Bayley, L., & Haynes, R. B. (2009). Accessing pre-appraised evidence: Fine-tuning the 5S model into a 6S model. *Evidence-Based Nursing, 12*(4), 99–101.

Dynamed. (2022). *Visceral Leishmaniasis*. [online] Dynamed. Accessed November 18, 2018, from https://www.dynamed.com/topics/dmp~AN~T113881

EBSCO Information Services. (2024). *Editorial Process | DynaMed Solutions | EBSCO*. [online] EBSCO. Accessed May 6, 2025, from https://www.ebsco.com/clinical-decisions/dynamed-solutions/about/evidence-based-process/editorial-process

European Union. (2022). *EU citizens: over half seek health information online*. [online] Eurostat. Accessed May 6, 2025, from https://ec.europa.eu/eurostat/web/products-eurostat-news/-/edn-20220406-1

Eysenbach, G. (2002). Infodemiology: The epidemiology of (mis)information. *The American Journal of Medicine, 113*(9), 763–765.

Eysenbach, G. (2006). Infodemiology: Tracking flu-related searches on the web for syndromic surveillance. *American Medical Informatics Association Annual Symposium Proceedings, 2006*, 244–248.

Eysenbach, G. (2009). Infodemiology and infoveillance: Framework for an emerging set of public health informatics methods to analyze search, communication and publication behavior on the Internet. *Journal of Medical Internet Research, 1*(1), e11.

References

Eysenbach, G. (2020). How to fight an infodemic: The four pillars of infodemic management. *Journal of Medical Internet Research, 22*(6), e21820.

Eysenbach, G., Powell, J., Kuss, O., et al. (2002). Empirical studies assessing the quality of health information for consumers on the World Wide Web: A systematic review. *JAMA, 287*(20), 2691–2700.

Fernandes, T., & Costa, R. (2013). As comunidades de Manguinhos na história das favelas no Rio de Janeiro. *Revista Tempo, 19*(34), 117–133.

Freire, P. (1987). *Pedagogy of the opressed*. Paz e Terra.

Fritsch, A., & Sigmund, H. (2016). Review platforms in hospitality. In R. Egger, I. Gula, & D. Walcher (Eds.), *Open tourism* (pp. 229–238). Springer.

Furlan, L., & Caramelli, B. (2021). The regrettable story of the "Covid Kit" and the "Early Treatment of Covid-19" in Brazil. *The Lancet Regional Health Americas, 4*, 100089.

Garbin, H. B., Pereira Neto, A., & Guilam, M. C. (2008). A internet, o paciente expert e a prática médica: uma análise bibliográfica. *Interface, 12*(26), 579–588.

Generalitat de Catalunya. (2024a). *Inici*. [online] Gencat.cat. Accessed May 6, 2025, from https://web.gencat.cat/ca/inici

Generalitat de Catalunya. (2024b). *Símptomes de la tuberculosi*. [online] Canal Salut. Accessed May 6, 2025, from https://canalsalut.gencat.cat/ca/salut-a-z/t/tuberculosi/simptomes/

Gonzalez-Argote, J. (2022). Effective communication and shared decision making: Theoretical approach from the doctor-patient relationship approach. *Seminars in Medical Writing and Education, 1*, 12.

Gouvernement du Québec. (2024). *Tuberculose*. [online] Gouvernement du Québec. Accessed May 6, 2025, from https://www.quebec.ca/sante/problemes-de-sante/a-z/tuberculose

Gouvernement du Québec. (2025). *Problèmes de santé de A à Z*. [online] Gouvernement du Québec. Accessed May 6, 2025, from https://www.quebec.ca/sante/problemes-de-sante/a-z

Higgins, J. P., & Green, S. (2008). *Cochrane Handbook for Systematic Reviews of Interventions* (Vol. 5). Hoboken, NJ: Wiley.

Kuenzel, U., Monga Sindeu, T., Schroth, S., et al. (2018). Evaluation of the quality of online information for patients with rare cancers: Thyroid cancer. *Journal of Cancer Education, 33*(5), 960–966.

Kwag, K. H., González-Lorenzo, M., Banzi, R., et al. (2016). Providing doctors with high-quality information: An updated evaluation of web-based point-of-care information summaries. *Journal of Medical Internet Research, 18*(1), e15.

Lévy, P. (2001). *Cyberculture*. University of Minnesota Press.

Liang, L. L., Kuo, H. S., Ho, H. J., et al. (2021). COVID-19 vaccinations are associated with reduced fatality rates: Evidence from cross-country quasi-experiments. *Journal of Global Health, 11*, 05019.

MedlinePlus. (2019a). *MedlinePlus*. [online] Medlineplus. Accessed May 6, 2025, from https://medlineplus.gov/spanish/

MedlinePlus. (2019b). *Tuberculosis*. [online] MedlinePlus. Accessed May 6, 2025, from https://medlineplus.gov/spanish/tuberculosis.html

Ministry of Health. (2022). *Tuberculose*. [online] Ministério da Saúde. Accessed May 6, 2025, from https://www.gov.br/saude/pt-br/assuntos/saude-de-a-a-z/t/tuberculose

Ministry of Health. (2023). *Leishmaniose Visceral*. [online] Ministry of Health. Accessed May 6, 2025, from https://www.gov.br/saude/pt-br/assuntos/saude-de-a-a-z/l/leishmaniose-visceral

Ministry of Health. (2024). *Boletim Epidemiológico - Tuberculose (2024) [Epidemiological Bulletin - Tuberculosis 2024]*. [online] Ministry of Health, Brasília, DF. Accessed May 3, 2025, from https://www.gov.br/aids/pt-br/central-de-conteudo/boletins-epidemiologicos/2024/boletim-epidemiologico-tuberculose-2024/view

Nadanovsky, P. (1999). Epidemiologia aplicada a clínica: um enfoque científico do uso da informação médica - Medicina Baseada em Evidência. *Estudos em Saúde Coletiva, 185*, 1–27.

National Health Service. (2019). *Health A-Z*. [online] NHS. Accessed May 6, 2025, from https://www.nhs.uk/conditions/

National Health Service. (2023). *Tuberculosis (TB)*. [online] NHS. Accessed May 6, 2025, from https://www.nhs.uk/conditions/tuberculosis-tb/

Paolucci, R. (2015). Methods for assessing the quality of information on health websites: a systematic review (2001-2014). 150 p. Dissertation (Master's in Health Information and Communication) - Postgraduate Program in Health Information and Communication, Oswaldo Cruz Foundation, Rio de Janeiro.

Paolucci, R. (2020). *Avaliação da qualidade da informação em sites de saúde: indicadores de acurácia baseada em evidência para tuberculose*. Oswaldo Cruz Foundation, Rio de Janeiro [Doctoral dissertation]. Accessed May 3, 2025, from https://www.arca.fiocruz.br/handle/icict/47262

Paolucci, R., Pereira, A., & Luzia, R. (2017). Avaliação da qualidade da informação em sites de tuberculose: análise de uma experiência participativa. *Saúde debate, 41*, 84–100.

Paolucci, R., & Pereira Neto, A. (2021). Methods for evaluating the quality of information on health websites: Systematic Review (2001-2014). *Latin American Journal of Development, 3*(3), 37–42.

Paolucci, R., Pereira Neto, A., & Nadanovsky, P. (2021). Avaliação da acurácia da informação em sites de saúde: métodos para construção de indicadores baseados em evidência [Evaluation of information accuracy in health sites: Methods for constructing evidence-based indicators]. *Em Questão, 27*(4), 137–188.

Paolucci, R., Pereira Neto, A., & Nadanovsky, P. (2022). Assessment of the quality of health information on the Internet: Evidence-based accuracy indicators for tuberculosis. *Saúde debate, 46*(135), 931–973.

Pariser, E. (2011). *The filter bubble: What the internet is hiding from you*. Penguin Press.

Passarelli-Araujo, H., Pott-Junior, H., Susuki, A. M., et al. (2022). The impact of COVID-19 vaccination on case fatality rates in a city in Southern Brazil. *American Journal of Infection Control, 50*(5), 491–496.

Peixoto, J. S. M., Soares, F. A., Brasil, S. S., et al. (2023). Práticas de ciência cidadã para promoção da saúde: o caso do Laboratório Internet, Saúde e Sociedade (LaISS) da Fiocruz. *Rev. cient. UEM, 4*(1), 166–169.

Pereira Neto, A., Ferreira, E., Barbosa, L., et al. (2023). Evaluation of the accuracy of the information on websites about visceral leishmaniasis: A strategy for countering information disorder. *Saúde debate, 47*(136), 126–140.

Pereira Neto, A., Lima, J. F., Barbosa, L., et al. (2019). Internet, Expert patient, and empowerment: Activity profiles in virtual communities of chronic kidney patients. In A. Pereira Neto & M. Flynn (Eds.), *Internet and health in Brazil: Challenges and trends* (pp. 87–111). Springer.

Pereira Neto, A., López, S. B., Almeida, J. A., et al. (2021). Assessment of the quality of information on breastfeeding sites: Notes on an experience. In P. Silva & D. Leite (Eds.), *Saúde coletiva: avanços e desafios para a integralidade do cuidado* (Vol. 3, pp. 114–127).

Pereira Neto, A., & Paolucci, R. (2019). Evaluation of the quality of health information on the internet: An analysis of Brazilian initiatives. In A. Pereira Neto & M. Flynn (Eds.), *Internet and health in Brazil: Challenges and trends* (pp. 181–209). Springer.

Pereira Neto, A. F., Paolucci, R., Daumas, R. P., et al. (2017). Avaliação participativa da qualidade da informação de saúde na internet: o caso de sites de dengue [Participatory evaluation of the quality of health information on the internet: The case of dengue sites]. *Ciência & Saúde Coletiva, 22*(6), 1955–1968.

Ryhänen, A. M., Rankinen, S., Siekkinen, M., et al. (2012). The impact of an empowering Internet-based Breast Cancer Patient Pathway programme on breast cancer patients' knowledge: A randomised control trial. *Patient Education and Counseling, 88*(2), 224–231.

Sackett, D. L., Rosenberg, W. M., Gray, J. A., et al. (1996). Evidence based medicine: What it is and what it isn't. *BMJ, 312*(7023), 71–72.

Silberg, W. M., Lundberg, G. D., & Musacchio, R. A. (1997). Assessing, controlling, and assuring the quality of medical information on the internet: Caveant Lector et Viewor—Let the reader and viewer beware. *JAMA, 277*(15), 1244–1245.

Stoll, M., Kerwer, M., Lieb, K., et al. (2022). Plain language summaries: A systematic review of theory, guidelines and empirical research. *PLoS One, 17*(6), e0268789.

Suarez-Lledo, V., & Alvarez-Galvez, J. (2021). Prevalence of health misinformation on social media: Systematic review. *Journal of Medical Internet Research, 23*(1), e17187.

Tangcharoensathien, V., Calleja, N., Nguyen, T., et al. (2020). Framework for managing the COVID-19 infodemic: Methods and results of an online, crowdsourced WHO technical consultation. *Journal of Medical Internet Research, 22*(6), e19659.

TB CARE I. (2014). *International Standards for Tuberculosis Care, Edition 3*. TB CARE I.

TB-CTA. (2006). *International Standards for Tuberculosis Care (ISTC)*. Tuberculosis Coalition for Technical Assistance (TB-CTA).

Tones, K. (2002). Health literacy: New wine in old bottles? *Health Education Research, 17*, 287–290.

Wang, X., & Cohen, R. A. (2023). *Health information technology use among adults: United States, July–December 2022*. [online] Centers for Disease Control and Prevention. US Department of Health and Human Services, Washington, DC. Accessed May 3, 2025, from https://www.cdc.gov/nchs/data/databriefs/db482.pdf

Waszak, P., Kasprzycka-Waszak, W., & Kubanek, A. (2018). The spread of medical fake news in social media – The pilot quantitative study. *Health Policy and Technology, 7*(2).

World Health Organization. (2020a). *Munich Security Conference*. [online] World Health Organization. Accessed May 3, 2025, from http://who.int/director-general/speeches/detail/munich-security-conference

World Health Organization. (2020b). *WHO: Health Assembly adopts resolution on the global response to COVID-19*. [online] Third World Network Berhad. Accessed May 12, 2025, from https://twn.my/title2/intellectual_property/info.service/2020/ip200509.htm

World Health Organization. (2025). *Tuberculosis*. [online] World Health Organization. Accessed May 6, 2025, from https://www.who.int/news-room/fact-sheets/detail/tuberculosis

Yang, Y., Hou, M., & Gong, X. (2022). Quality assessment of hypertension treatment–related information on WeChat: Cross-sectional study. *Journal of Medical Internet Research, 24*(10), e38567.

Zhang, X. (2022). Incremental innovation: Long-term impetus for design business creativity. *Sustainability, 14*(22), 14697.

Zhang, Y., Sun, Y., & Xie, B. (2015). Quality of health information for consumers on the web: A systematic review of indicators, criteria, tools, and evaluation results. *Journal of the Association for Information Science and Technology, 66*(10), 2071–2084.

Chapter 3
Digital Literacy Against Disinformation: Vital Pedagogical Practice for All of Us, Forever

Abstract The new information and communication technologies are changing society from an economic, social, and political point of view. Infinite opportunities are offered through these technologies which, in turn, become an integral part of our daily lives. Citizens need to be digitally literate to know how to use and take advantage of them. This chapter presents the "State of the Art" on the definition of "digital literacy" using bibliographic reviews published in recent years on the subject. It notes that the studies made on "digital literacy" between 2020 and 2025 do not associate this pedagogical practice as one of the ways to fight disinformation. It highlights the role that the critical and creative use of information obtained and shared in digital media can play in fighting health disinformation on the Internet. It proposes that "digital literacy" becomes a permanent pedagogical practice, as it is necessary and vital for all of us, throughout our lives.

Keywords Digital literacy · Digital inclusion · Information society

3.1 Introduction

I was born in 1958 in the city of Rio de Janeiro, Brazil. My parents had married 8 years earlier and went to live in a remote neighborhood in the center of the city of Rio de Janeiro. My mother was a housewife. My father, a civil engineer. We had means, as we lived in a house of our own with a private phone, which was in the hallway. The device was black, heavy, and large with a crank outside. On the phone, there was no way to dial or enter the number to be called. To use it, my mother turned this crank and took the headset off the hook. A telephone operator answered a few seconds later and said "Good morning!" Then my mother would say, "Hello? This is Sonia!" And the operator replied: "Good morning, Mrs. Sonia! How are you?" And my mother would say: "I'm fine... and you, Luiza?" My mother recognized the operator's voice. At that time, there were only two operators that carried out that activity in the neighborhood where we lived. An animated chat would start between the two until my mother asked, "Can you call my mother?" Luiza already knew that my grandmother lived in a neighborhood located at the other end of the city. Then Luiza replied: "I'll try Mrs. Sonia, wait a little, please." Then my mother would thank her and hang up the phone. A few minutes later, the phone would ring in my house. My mother would answer and hear Luiza say, with great delight: "Mrs. Sonia, I managed ... you can talk to your mother!" This was how people spoke on the phone in the late 1950s in the elite homes of Brazil. This reality was similar to that of other wealthy families residing in other regions of the planet at the same time. Having a phone was a privilege for a few. Talking on the phone was no easy task. It required this informal contact and an etiquette of its own.

Several authors have written about the history of the telephone, exploring its technological development, social impact, and the characters involved in its creation and popularization. The book by Fischer (1992) became a reference work on the subject.

According to Fischer (1992), the history of the telephone began when Alexander Graham Bell, the inventor of this technology, called his friend Thomas Watson. Thus began a process of technological change that transformed everyday life and human relations. It took the telephone a few decades to become a popular vehicle of communication. In developed countries, this vehicle of communication was restricted to the economic elite until the end of the Second World War.

Fischer (1992) analyzes how the telephone allowed people to keep contact with distant family members and friends and contributed to the transformation of the dynamics of personal, economic, cultural, and social relationships. He highlights the contrast in phone adoption between users in rural areas and inhabitants of urban regions. Fischer (1992) also reveals how the telephone created etiquette norms on how to start and end calls correctly. The author discusses the role of women as telephone operators. He highlights how the telephone gradually became a domestic tool, often associated with maintaining family relationships. The case of the communication between my mother and the telephone operator illustrates this idea well, especially because my mother intended to talk to my grandmother and thus strengthen her family ties, make requests, and share information. The author also points out that in the 1960s, the telephone became popular and ceased to be a technological curiosity to become an indispensable tool in everyday life, especially in developed countries. In more remote regions or in developing countries, popularization took even longer, extending until the end of the twentieth century.

The case of Brazil can serve as an example in this regard. Until the 1970s, having a phone at home was a privilege for a few, even in urban areas. My family was one of the few to enjoy this advantage from the 1960s. In rural areas of Brazil, access to the telephone was almost non-existent. Starting from the 1980s, the federal government began to invest in telecommunications infrastructure. Thus, the number of telephone lines increased significantly. However, the service was still expensive and bureaucratic. It was common to have long waiting lists for the installation of telephone lines. Many families still depended on public telephone booths (Feldmann & Belluzzo, 2011). As the infrastructure was obsolete, there were few telephone lines available in the market. Thus, the demand for telephone lines outstripped the supply.

3.1 Introduction

For a long time, a telephone line would cost so much that it could serve as part of the payment for automobiles and real estate. In 1972, the Federal Government of Brazil created "Telebrás": a state-owned company that became responsible for unifying and expanding telephone services in the country. It did not have the necessary level of investment and its objectives were not reached. In 1998, this company was privatized. This initiative attracted foreign investment and allowed the modernization of infrastructure, but also led to increased charges and market concentration in the hands of a few foreign companies (Feldmann & Belluzzo, 2011). This process of internationalization of fixed telephony can be observed in other regions of the planet (Castells, 1996).

In developing countries, the telephone has ceased to be a product for few only since the 1990s. In the developed countries, popularization has been related to the 1960s. Therefore, it took practically 100 years for the telephone to leave Bell's hands and reach the homes of all of us.

As we mentioned in the first chapter of this book, at the end of the twentieth century, while the telephone was becoming popular, a technological innovation began to take place: the mobile phone. An innovation that has had profound impacts on society, economy, and culture. Let's take a look at its history.

In April 1973, Martin Cooper, the Motorola engineer who invented the mobile phone, made his first call using the *Motorola DynaTAC 8000X*.

The *Motorola DynaTAC 8000X* was a revolutionary device for its time. It looks rudimentary compared to contemporary cell phones. *DynaTAC* was basically a portable phone, very expensive and only capable of making phone calls. Nothing further.

The first device to be considered a *smartphone* was the *IBM Simon*, launched in 1994 in partnership with *BellSouth*. It had a touchscreen (monochrome). The device could make and receive phone calls and had other functions such as calendar, contact list, notepad, and email. It was possible to install additional applications, albeit to a limited extent. It was accompanied by a *stylus* to facilitate the user's interaction with the screen. It was big and heavy compared to current *smartphones*. Its battery only lasted an hour. It was not widely adopted due to its high cost ($899 at the time). However, the *IBM Simon smartphone* is considered a milestone in the history of mobile communication devices by bringing to the phone functions that were performed only on the computer (Mercer, 2006). It was only in the 2000s, with the launch of the *iPhone* and *Android*, that *smartphones* began to become popular.

Castells et al. (2007) published a book that analyzes the impact of mobile communication devices on society. It demonstrates how they have transformed social, economic, and political life in different parts of the world. The book highlights the rapid adoption of mobile communication. As we mentioned above, the iPhone and the Android were launched in the year 2000. They started the diffusion of mobile technologies with different functions. Thus, it took only a little more than 20 years for *smartphones* to be present in the lives of the majority of the planet's population and to redefine the way in which we interact, work, and organize ourselves. As we mentioned earlier, with the telephone, it took about 100 years. With the smartphone it took just over 20 years. A very fast, profound, and definitive change.

Castells et al. (2007) admit that cell phones facilitate communication but also bring new challenges, such as technological addiction, the erosion of face-to-face interactions, and the loss of privacy. For them, mobile communication is at the heart of the transformation to a "networked society," where digital connections are as important as physical interactions. Castells et al. (2007) demonstrate that mobile communication is becoming increasingly integrated into everyday life, with profound implications for the future of society. Mobile communication is also seen as a powerful tool for democratization, enabling citizens to actively participate in the political process and report abuses of power.

Turkle (2011) analyzes how the use of mobile devices is transforming human relationships and how one person connects with another. In his view, information and communication technologies are leading us to replace authentic human connections with superficial interactions that use machines. According to him, this practice can cause a feeling of loneliness regardless of the person being connected.

The changes introduced by new information and communication technologies through mobile devices are therefore noticeable in different dimensions of human life. They have significantly modified labor relations. The operator who made the phone call with my mother no longer exists! There is no longer a banker behind a bank counter to check your signature and cash a check. We don't need to go to the bank to pay a bill. Today, payments are made through applications available on mobile phones. The librarian who guided us in the bibliographic research is no longer in the library. From home, at the distance of a touch, we visit libraries in different parts of the world and access international bibliographic databases, often free of charge. The election and submission of the income statement are carried out through digital media. In the first case, the results are almost immediate, and fraud, very common in paper voting times, is avoided. When filling out my income statement last year, I was surprised by the fact that the Federal Revenue system makes all my data available in the spreadsheet as soon as it includes my number in the "Individual Taxpayer Registry" (CPF). The restructuring of the production base is visible when we get on a bus, and we no longer find the exchanger: a professional who sold the urban bus ticket and gave change if the amount paid in cash by the user was higher than the price of the ticket. Today, there is a magnetic card that allows the user to get on the bus and make their trip. The restructuring of the productive base is not the topic we will analyze and discuss in this chapter. However, it is something to bear in mind (Temelkova, 2023).

3.2 Digital Exclusion

Throughout this chapter, and all through this book, we are insisting on the idea that the changes promoted by New Information and Communication Technologies have occurred in all spheres of social life at an astonishing speed.

However, not everyone has signed up for this digital world in the same way. Some are—and continue to be—digitally divided. Digital Divide: What's that?

3.2 Digital Exclusion

The digital divide, also known as the "digital exclusion" or "digital breach," referred, until some time ago, to the inequality encompassing certain people when wanting to have access to information and communication technologies (ICTs). In that context, the digitally excluded was a citizen who did not have access to the Internet. He experienced this condition because he did not have the financial resources to acquire a computer. Added to this is the fact that access is made through a cable. This technical aspect prevented access from being made possible, especially in low-income communities or in those located in regions far enough from urban centers for the cable to reach, and where it could even be intercepted by militias or drug traffickers. The digitally excluded person was, to a large extent, a socially excluded person. This reality has not changed in some regions of the planet.

The International Telecommunication Union (ITU) is a United Nations (UN) agency specializing in issues related to information and communication technologies (ICTs). ITU collects and disseminates data and conducts research around the world to monitor growth and digital transformation.

The ITU estimates that approximately 5.5 billion people (68% of the world's population) were using the Internet in 2024. This represents an increase from 2019, when it indicated that 1.3 billion people were *online*. Despite this growth, the ITU estimates that 2.6 billion people do not have access to the Internet. The African continent concentrates the largest number of countries where less than 42% of the population has access to the Internet (ITU, 2025). In this case, the countries of the sub-Saharan region stand out due to the combination of historical, economic, social, and geographical factors. In this region, the electrical and telecommunications infrastructure is insufficient or poorly distributed. In addition, extreme weather conditions have damaged existing infrastructure. This problem becomes even more serious in rural areas, deserts, and forests. It is worth remembering that the installation costs are high and that the population lives with high levels of poverty and is immersed in illiteracy and in a context of strong political instability (Jafar et al., 2024). In this case, South Sudan stands out, where only 9.7% of the population has access to the Internet.

Shanahan and Bahia (2024) published *The State of Mobile Internet Connectivity 2024* by the GSMA (Global System for Mobile Communications Association): an international organization that represents the interests of mobile operators and companies in the mobile technology ecosystem around the world. With the data obtained, the authors conclude that:

> Sub-Saharan Africa remains the region with the lowest connectivity levels and largest coverage gap. Connectivity is highest in Southern and Western Africa at around 30%, and lowest in Central Africa at 19%. Central Africa also has the largest coverage gap, at 34% […]. Eastern Africa has the largest usage gap within the region, at 68% (Shanahan & Bahia, 2024, p. 10)

On the other hand, data from the "International Telecommunication Union" reveal that more than 42% of the population is connected. The arrival of the wireless access and the fall in the price of mobile devices made it possible for those people to have a mobile device in their hands.

Recent data signal this reality. In Brazil, the "Regional Center for Studies for the Development of the Information Society" (Cetic.br) monitors the adoption of information and communication technologies (ICT). Since 2005, it has conducted an annual survey on the use of information and communication technologies in households. In 2022, Cetic.br carried out another survey on access to Information and Communication Technologies in Brazilian households (Brazilian Network Information Center, 2023). The results indicate that 84% of Brazilian households have access to the Internet. However, the possession of a computer in households remains a characteristic associated with the location and socioeconomic condition of the user. This is because more than half of the households in the D and E classes do not have a computer (56%). In addition, about one in ten Brazilians, from D and E classes, aged 10 years or older, has never accessed the Internet. In Brazil, this represents approximately 20 million individuals. Among those who have never used the Internet are citizens aged 60 or over (42%), those in classes D and E (22%), and those who have studied until elementary school (18%) (Brazilian Network Information Center, 2023).

Thus, the data presented above give testimony that the digitally excluded individual is not just that citizen who resides in areas where there is no connectivity. The digitally excluded individual is also the person who has a smartphone and knows how to access, produce, or share information through digital media. He doesn't know, however, how to make a bank transfer. He doesn't know how to enroll his son in school. He doesn't know how to take a picture with his phone and send it to someone. He doesn't know how to tell a false information from a true one! He does not know how to identify fraudulent information. This group is still mostly made up of individuals with low purchasing power and poor education. In general terms, a large part of the digitally excluded population currently lives in urban centers in peripheral and impoverished neighborhoods of the planet. They are also socially excluded.

The same report indicated that the lack of skill was the reason that led many users to not use their cell phones or computers despite having these technological devices. I myself, from the top of my 66 years, need to learn how to deal with these new information and communication technologies. The description I made of my youth at the beginning of this chapter gives testimony that reality has changed a lot. Every day, a new function appears on mobile phones. If I face this difficulty, what about people with poor education? What about people who have cognitive, visual, or motor difficulties?

Thus, the access, use, and appropriation of information available and shared in digital media have become an indispensable part of all our lives. We cannot imagine a world without access to and ownership of the functions and facilities available through new information and communication technologies. I have a hard time putting myself in the shoes of someone who owns a mobile device but doesn't know how to take advantage of it. Information and communication technologies are no longer just a complementary tool to our communication. New ICT has become a primary means to carry out our daily activities, ranging from basic things like talking and messaging to more sophisticated activities such as getting a job or learning something new.

3.2 Digital Exclusion

Those who do not know how to deal with these ICTs will find it very difficult to carry out many social and economic activities. Silva (2022) estimates that:

> [...] 85% of the professions that will exist in 2030 do not yet exist. This statement is a warning of the constant changes, which for some may be a window of opportunity and for others a real difficulty in adapting. (Silva, 2022, p. 3)

For this reason, it has become imperative to learn how to deal with these technologies. Basic digital skills are needed for each of us to be able to enter this new world: The Digital World. We need to be digitally literate!

The term "digital literacy" was first conceived by Paul Gilster (1997). He defined "digital literacy" as the ability to understand and use information in multiple formats available through new information and communication technologies (Gilster, 1997). For him, "digital literacy" is closely linked to individual skills in accessing, evaluating, and managing information.

Since Gilster (1997) first formulated the definition of this concept, many authors have presented different versions of this term. They also presented different views on the purposes of "digital literacy." We will present, below, the "State of the Art" of the bibliographic production on "digital literacy."

3.2.1 State of the Art

This expression is used to refer to research that maps the academic production on a topic. As stated by Teixeira (2023), the "State of the Art" studies are:

> [...] dedicated to identifying, mapping, describing and analyzing—on multiple dimensions and aspects, according to the interest of the investigation—the set of research developed in a given area of knowledge. Therefore, they are studies dedicated to investigating the evolutionary dynamics of research within an area, in a given region (country, continent, etc.), according to the time frame defined for the survey of works belonging to the scope of interest. (Teixeira, 2023, p. 6)

In this chapter, we will analyze the bibliographic reviews on "digital literacy" published between 2020 and 2025. For this purpose, we used *Google Scholar* using the expression "digital literacy review" in the search engine. Six articles were found.

We will initially see the institutional origin of its authors, the methods adopted, and the objectives of each of these studies. Next, we will analyze the place that the authors give to this pedagogical practice as an alternative to fight disinformation.

The first article was published in 2020 by three researchers from the Fiji National University and the University of the South Pacific (USP), in the Fiji Islands (Reddy et al., 2020). The authors report that this is an "Integrative *Literature Review.*"

According to Whittemore and Knafl (2005), an "Integrative Literature Review" should explain the search route of the articles and cite the articles that served as a source for the conclusions presented. Snyder (2019) states that an "Integrative Literature Review" should explain the way in which the articles were selected. Reddy et al. (2020) did not make clear the methodological paths taken by them or the results achieved. Despite this, according to *Google Scholar*, this article was the most cited among the six that make up our sample. Until March 2025, 465 authors mentioned this article in their respective analyses.

In the abstract of this article, Reddy et al. (2020) state that:

> Information and communication technologies (ICT) along with the internet have fueled advancements and growth in banking, transportation, economics, and most of all in education in the 21st century. The 21st century citizens are provided with new opportunities that have been created with the advancement of ICT. Hence, individuals need a wide range of abilities, competencies, and skills to adapt to the technological era. This paper provides a literature review of the growing importance of ICT, its wide array of usage, and its influence on various facets of people's daily lives. (Reddy et al., 2020, p. 1)

The second bibliographic study was published 2 years later by Peng and Yu (2022) from the Beijing Language and Culture University in Beijing, China. The authors followed the guidelines and performed *The Preferred Reporting Items for Systematic Review and Meta-Analysis—PRISMA*. They conducted bibliographic research on the Web of Science: an important international bibliographic base. The bibliographic analysis by Peng and Yu (2022) was performed using 20 titles. Its abstract states that:

> [...] this paper focused on the definition of digital literacy; the factors affecting students' digital literacy (age, gender, family socioeconomic status, and parent's education level); the relationship between students' digital literacy and their self-control, technostress, and engagement; and the three approaches to gauge the level of students' digital literacy. (Peng and Yu 2022, p. 1).

The third study found was published by four authors from institutions located in different parts of the world (Tinmaz et al., 2022), namely: "Woosong University," in Daejeon—South Korea; "University of Economic Studies,", in Bucharest—Romania and the "School of Management,", in Abu Dhabi—United Arab Emirates. In this case, the authors mentioned the bibliographic databases that were searched and the search route used. Forty-three (43) articles served as the basis for the conclusions presented. Its abstract states that "The purpose of this study is to discover the main themes and categories of the research studies regarding digital literacy" (Tinmaz et al., 2022, p. 1).

The fourth article was published by six researchers from different institutions, all located in Italy (Campanozzi et al., 2023). To carry out this literature review, the authors searched three important international bibliographic databases, namely: *PubMed*, *Scopus,* and *Web of Science* (WoS). In doing so, they reached 37 titles published between January 2011 and October 2022. Its objective is "to define, through a review of the literature of the past 10 years, the extent of the impact of digital literacy on access to telemedicine services" (Campanozzi et al., 2023, p. 2).

The fifth paper was published by researchers at Korea University in Seoul (Ban et al., 2024). They used six databases (PubMed, Embase, CINAHL, RISS, KISS, and DBpia) and Google Scholar. In doing so, they reached 32 titles published between 2006 and 2023. The study objective was

3.2 Digital Exclusion

> To elucidate the concept of digital health literacy by delineating its primary dimensions, origins and effects. Through this clarification, we seek to augment our understanding of the contemporary use of the concept of digital health literacy. (Ban et al., 2024, p. 1)

The last study we used in this chapter was published in 2025 by five researchers (Zhong et al., 2025). Four of them work at "Southwest University" in Chongqing, China and one at "Seventh Middle School" in Guizhou, China.

Its abstract states that:

> The purpose of this study is to analyse the current research status, hotspots and development trends of teachers' digital literacy in China. The article uses Citespace to visualize and analyse 1,129 relevant Chinese literature published between 2007 and 2024 in China Knowledge Network CNKI. (Zhong et al., 2025, p. 3)

Thus, the survey we carried out seems quite comprehensive to us. The six bibliographic analyses on "digital literacy," which will be analyzed below, were published by researchers from important academic institutions in the world, in renowned journals of international circulation. The authors followed, in general, the methodological principles for carrying out bibliographic analyses, as they presented the documentary bases used, the paths adopted, and the results obtained (Snyder 2019).

The sample period, restricted to 5 years (2020/2025), is justified due to the superabundance of information, one corrects the other does not, called "infodemic" (Eysenbach, 2020), evident during the COVID-19 pandemic. Thus, we start from the hypothesis that academic production produced in this period would establish a relationship between "digital literacy" and the confrontation with disinformation.

The objective of this chapter is to verify if the studies on "digital literacy," between 2020 and 2025, understand that this pedagogical practice can be seen as one of the ways to combat health disinformation. The concerns that guide this chapter accompany the reflections introduced by Eysenbach (2020) when he proposed an "infodemic" management strategy as follows:

> I am positing four pillars of infodemic management: (1) information monitoring (infoveillance); (2) *building eHealth Literacy and science literacy capacity* [emphasis added]; (3) encouraging knowledge refinement and quality improvement processes such as fact checking and peer-review; and (4) accurate and timely knowledge translation, minimizing distorting factors such as political or commercial influences. (Eysenbach, 2020, p. 1)

According to Eysenbach (2020), "digital literacy" should guide users to discern true information from false information.

The hope we had when starting this investigation was that we would find studies that had made this association. After all, Campanozzi et al. (2023, p. 2) stated that they would analyze "the extent of the impact of digital literacy." The fight against disinformation is, as far as we see, one of the possible impacts. Ban et al. (2024), in turn, aimed to outline the dimensions, origins, and effects of "digital literacy." One of the effects, in our view, is to contribute to the fight against disinformation.

3.3 Digital Literacy and the Fight Against Disinformation

We will see below if the studies found in the bibliographic analyses that make up our chapter established the association between "digital literacy" and the fight against disinformation. Our analysis will follow the chronological order of publication.

The first study we analyzed was published by Reddy et al. (2020).

The authors understand that "digital literacy" is an essential competency in the digital age. For them, the development of "digital literacy" faces significant challenges, such as the digital divide and the lack of standardization in the pedagogical process. According to them, collaborative efforts between governments, educational institutions, and communities are needed to ensure that all individuals have the necessary skills to fully participate in the digital society (Reddy et al., 2020).

The articles analyzed by these authors revealed that a digitally literate citizen is someone who has sufficient knowledge in the management of new information and communication technologies to be able to use them efficiently and effectively. To do so, he must have a variety of skills (technical and cognitive) to disseminate, locate digital information "using well-designed search strategies and *critically evaluate it and judge the quality*" [emphasis added] (Reddy et al., 2020, p. 83).

They define the digitally literate as someone who is able to critically evaluate and judge the quality of information. When detailing the "Information Literacy," the authors state that:

> Using digital technology to find, locate, analyse and synthesise resources, *evaluating the credibility of these resources* [emphasis added] appropriate citation techniques, abiding the legal and ethical issues surrounding the use of these resources and formulating research questions in an accurate, effective and efficient manner. (Reddy et al., 2020, p. 84).

Thus, the article by Reddy et al. (2020) does not explicitly associate digital literacy with fighting disinformation.

The second study we analyzed was published by Peng and Yu in 2022. The authors begin their bibliographic analysis by admitting that the results of COVID-19 have terribly affected different sectors, including education. According to them: "Plenty of students had to leave their school and stay at home. The educational sectors turned to online education immediately to fight against the pandemic crisis" (Peng & Yu, 2022, p. 1).

Peng and Yu (2022) complement this idea by concluding that "digital literacy" is not a new term. They state that:

> In a nutshell, some of the definitions only place emphasis on digital skills, while others focus on the multidimensional concept. It is of vital significance to increase both the basic digital skills and those skills by which people understand and use the online content. (Peng & Yu, 2022, p. 2)

They analyzed 20 studies that evaluated the factors that interfered with students' "digital literacy" during the pandemic. The 20 studies analyzed by Peng and Yu (2022) indicate four factors: Age, gender, family socioeconomic status, and educational background. They concluded this study by stating that:

3.3 Digital Literacy and the Fight Against Disinformation

Students' digital literacy could affect students' self-control, technostress, and engagement in learning. Students' high level of digital literacy could significantly enhance their self-control and engagement in learning and reduce their technostress in class. (Peng & Yu, 2022, p. 6)

We were surprised that the 20 studies did not take into account the informational dispute about preventive procedures that characterized that moment in our recent history. A dispute that must have interfered with the students' self-control and technostress.

The third bibliographic analysis we observed was also published in 2022 (Tinmaz et al., 2022). In it, the authors concluded that "digital literacy" is "the human proficiencies to live, learn and work in the current digital society" (Tinmaz et al., 2022, p. 5). The same authors came to the conclusion that digital literacy must guide a person or society when interacting with digital technologies so they can know how to access, evaluate, and/or create information (Tinmaz et al., 2022).

Thus, the word 'assessment' suggests that the users make an assessment of the information they receive and search for. This may be an indication that some of the 43 articles analyzed by them have been concerned with the problem of information quality and its necessary evaluation.

Tinmaz et al. (2022) identified only three studies that suggest an approximation between "digital literacy" and coping with disinformation. The first one to be mentioned was *DigComp*.

Whereas digital thinking was observed to be mostly related with critical thinking and computational thinking, DigComp connects it with critical thinking, creativity, and innovation, on the one hand, and researchers highlight fake news, misinformation, cybersecurity, and echo chambers as exponents of digital thinking, on the other hand […] (Tinmaz et al., 2022, p. 12).

The "European Digital Competence Framework for Citizens" (*DigComp*) developed by the European Commission recommends eight levels of (digital) skills and abilities necessary for employment, personal development, and social inclusion (Carretero Gomez et al., 2017). These eight levels of competencies and skills range from information seeking, online interaction and sharing to the creation and development of digital materials, data protection and privacy, and problem solving (critical and innovative use of technology). None of the eight steps mention, the necessary qualification of the user to discern the right from the doubtful and identify fraudulent information.

The studies by Sulzer (2018) and Puig et al. (2021) are the ones that present a critical thinking on the subject.

Sulzer (2018) suggests a "(Re)conceptualizing digital literacies." According to him, the 2016 election in the USA revealed the deficiencies in the traditional digital literacy that prioritizes the mastering of technical skills rather than socio-political analysis. Trump's campaign and amplification of disinformation suggest a redefinition of "digital literacy." In his view, this pedagogical practice must take into account the power structures inherent to the sources of information. Therefore, "digital literacy" would no longer be a practice associated with individual competence. In this sense, the author states: "Thus, individuals entering into the social atmosphere of digital environments should be keenly aware that such social situations likely include entities (e.g., bots or actual people) with ulterior motives" (Sulzer, 2018, p. 64).

The third text was mentioned by Tinmaz et al. (2022) and was published by Puig et al. (2021). They explicitly mention the theme/problem of disinformation. Puig et al. (2021) start from the assumption that: "fake news covering all aspects of the pandemic spread rapidly through social media, creating confusion and disinformation" (Puig et al., 2021, p. 1).

The authors suggest that "critical thinking" be included in the practices of "digital literacy." Thus, students will become active citizens who will know how to deal with socio-scientific information and will be able to make decisions that affect their lives. According to them, the way science is taught in schools continues to be more oriented towards "what to think rather than to how to think."

Puig et al. (2021) conclude this study by stating that:

> This result highlights the importance of health literacy and its interdependence with CT development [...]. If we want to prepare students to develop CT in order to face real/false news spread by social media, we need to engage them in deep epistemic assessment, namely in the critical analysis of the content, the source, procedures and evidence behind the claims, apart from other tasks. (Puig et al., 2021, p. 8)

Thus, only 1 of the 43 articles analyzed by Tinmaz et al. (2022) included a dimension that takes into account confronting disinformation in the practices of "digital literacy."

The fourth literature review we analyzed assumes that health care in the third millennium is largely provided through systems involving the use of technological devices and services, particularly in telemedicine. (Campanozzi et al., 2023). The authors understand that users must be digitally literate for these services to be adequately offered. Campanozzi et al. (2023) conducted a review of academic literature in 37 articles to verify whether the user's level of "digital literacy" interferes with access to telemedicine services. They conclude this study by stating that:

> From this we can see that digital literacy programs are much more than teaching how to become familiar with the technological tools. In fact, making people digitally literate is primarily about teaching them to become aware of the scope and limitations of technological tools in the service of digital health. (Campanozzi et al., 2023, p. 4)

Campanozzi et al. (2023) were not concerned with the relationship between "digital literacy" and misinformation. For this reason, this topic/problem was not addressed in this study.

The fifth literature review was published by Ban et al. (2024). The objective of this study was to elucidate the concept of "digital literacy" in health, outlining its primary dimensions, origins, and effects. Through this clarification, the authors intend to improve the understanding of the contemporary use of the concept of digital health literacy.

3.3 Digital Literacy and the Fight Against Disinformation

Ban et al. (2024) present a brief history of the "digital literacy" concept, highlighting the specificity of health. In this article, Ban et al. (2024) present a table in which they offer a list of 13 authors who presented their respective definitions of "digital literacy" in health from 2006.

Two of them (Paige et al., 2018; Yoon, 2020) mention that the digitally literate must be able to "locate, understand, exchange and *evaluate* [emphasis added] health information" or to know "to use digital technology to find, *evaluate* [emphasis added] and communicate health-related information" (Ban et al., 2024, p. 5). The evaluation is a fundamental condition for the user to be able to discern the correct information from the fraudulent one, made available to cause damage.

The framework built by Ban et al. (2024) presents only one title that included the issue of disinformation in the definition of "digital literacy." It is the paper by Bodie and Dutta (2008). Ban et al. (2024) states that:

> […] High health literacy is not just the ability to use the Internet to find answers to health-related questions. […] It also entails the ability to understand the information found, […] *evaluate the veracity of this information*, […] *discern the quality of different websites* (emphasis added) […] and use quality information to make informed decisions about health. (Ban et al., 2024, p. 5)

We could summarize the ideas presented by Ban et al. (2024), stating that the digitally literate would be someone with three skills. One would have a technical character. With it, the user would be able to navigate using the different interfaces and information and communication technologies. Another would imply a critical sensitivity. Thus, the user could discern false information from the true. He should also have the interactive ability to communicate dexterously on different platforms. Finally, he should reveal the autonomy to make decisions independently. All this is aimed at concrete actions that change reality! In this regard, at the conclusion of their study, Ban et al. (2024) state that:

> Digital health literacy is here defined as the capacity to translate health knowledge acquired from digital environments into actions […]. (Ban et al., 2024, p. 13)

"Digital literacy" that followed these principles could empower the patient, reduce health disparities through Digital Health devices, and generate positive health outcomes. The risk caused by disinformation is also mentioned by the authors.

The sixth study we analyzed was written by Zhong et al. (2025). They carried out the most complete bibliographic analysis among those analyzed by us in this chapter. They handled more than a thousand titles published in China alone between 2007 and 2024.

They built several statistical tables. One demonstrates the evolution of academic production on "digital literacy" over time, and another presents a graph with the institutional origin of the authors.

It can be observed, that the association between "digital literacy" and disinformation was not identified in this broad bibliographic survey carried out by Zhong et al. (2025). The concern of these authors is different. They make this vision clear by stating that:

With the popularization of the Internet of Things and Artificial Intelligence and the rapid progress of digital technology, digital literacy not only affects individual learning and work efficiency, but also largely determines the economic competitiveness and social progress of a country and region. (Zhong et al., 2025, p. 4)

The results of the bibliographic analysis that we present in this chapter lead us to conclude that the investigations carried out on "digital literacy" did not realize that this pedagogical practice can be one of the ways to face disinformation.

This is not the perception of the World Health Organization (WHO).

Borges do Nascimento et al. (2022) published a systematic review in the "Bulletin of the World Health Organization" with the objective of identifying the challenges and opportunities presented to face health disinformation in the context of the COVID-19 pandemic. The scientific literature analyzed by these authors indicates that:

The most negative consequences of health misinformation are the increase of misleading or incorrect interpretations of available evidence, impact on mental health, misallocation of health resources and an increase in vaccination hesitancy. (Borges Do Nascimento et al., 2022, p. 544)

At the conclusion of this systematic review, the authors suggest that:

Multisectoral actions to counteract infodemics and health misinformation are needed, including developing legal policies, creating and promoting awareness campaigns, improving health-related content in mass media and *increasing people's digital and health literacy*. [emphasis added] (Borges Do Nascimento et al., 2022, p. 544)

The question now is: How to make someone digitally literate, keeping in mind the need to train them to have a critical awareness of the information received and shared in digital media?

This year, a systematic review was published by three researchers from the University of Extremadura in Caceres, Spain. Valverde-Berrocoso et al. (2025). They present an educational approach they consider appropriate, which is made up of three items, namely:

(a) A didactic approach with a broad vision of the disinformation phenomenon that enhances critical thinking, generates information production experiences and promotes attitudes compatible with a civic education; (b) Initial and ongoing teacher training that fosters the development of media and information literacy and digital competence; and (c) The development of interdisciplinary education and communication teams for research and teaching. (Valverde-Berrocoso et al., 2025, p. 103)

The European Commission published in 2022 *Guidelines for Teachers and Educators on Tackling Disinformation and Promoting Digital Literacy Through Education and Training*. It meets "a clear demand for strengthening the role of education and training when it comes to promoting digital literacy and tackling disinformation" (European Commission, 2022, p. 6).

Its goal is:

[…] to provide teachers and educators with learning objectives, pedagogical practices and hands-on activities in one user-friendly document focusing on what has been proven to work in classrooms and offering new ideas aimed to inspire teachers and young minds. (European Commission, 2022, p. 6).

The "Guideline" provides educators with practical tools. Thus, they will know how to combat disinformation and strengthen digital literacy in classrooms, preparing students to critically navigate the digital environment.

The "Guideline" has four objectives:

1. Providing insight and useful knowledge about the dynamics and manifestations of *disinformation* [emphasis added], as well as the defining characteristics of credible information.
2. Fostering an understanding of how digital literacy can be achieved.
3. Sharing information on how to use digital technologies critically and responsibly.
4. Providing insight into how students can be assessed regarding their competences in the field of digital literacy. (European Commission, 2022, p. 9)

The *Guidelines for Teachers and Educators on Tackling Disinformation and Promoting Digital Literacy Through Education and Training* seems to be the most complete document produced by a government agency aimed at training educators that associates "digital literacy" with combating disinformation.

In our view, the integration of "digital literacy" into educational systems as a strategy to combat disinformation is not simple. It is not enough to add new subjects or tools to your resume. This initiative requires a fundamental rethinking of how education is delivered and experienced. Class can't be more like it was 60 years ago. In the Information Society, teachers continue to play a key role. They remain the key enablers of learning.

For this reason, it is essential to provide educators with the training and resources necessary to effectively incorporate "digital literacy" into their teaching practices. This includes not only technical skills but also an understanding of the cultural and critical dimensions of information obtained and shared in digital media. The syllabus should be designed to reflect these dimensions, ensuring that students develop a holistic understanding of digital tools and their social and political implications. "Digital literacy" must be present from elementary school to higher education. It should be seen as an ongoing process that evolves along with technological progress.

3.4 Digital Literacy Against Disinformation: A Vital Pedagogical Practice for All, Forever

This is the title of this chapter. Let us see why.

Martin and Grudziecki (2006) propose, in their article, "levels" or steps for the development of "digital literacy."

The first level would be "Digital Competence." This is the moment when the user acquires the manual skills and fundamental cognitive skills to master the different possibilities of use and appropriation that digital technologies offer. In addition, they state that:

> Individuals or groups draw upon digital competence as is appropriate to their life situation, and return to gain more as new challenges are presented by the life situation. (Martin & Grudziecki, 2006, p. 255).

The second level would be "Digital Use." It corresponds to the moment when the user takes advantage of information and communication technologies. This can be observed, for example, when a mother manages to enroll her child on the website of the city hall of her city, or when a young person enrolls and attends an *online* course, or buys a product over the Internet.

> In order to complete the task or to solve the problem, the individual identifies a competence requirement. He/she may then acquire the needed digital competence through whatever learning process is available and preferred. He/she can then make an appropriate use of the acquired digital competence. The informed uses of digital competence within life-situations are termed here digital usages. These involve using digital tools to seek, find and process information, and then to develop a product or solution addressing the task or problem. This outcome will itself be the trigger for further action in the life context. (Martin & Grudziecki, 2006, p. 255)

The third level is "Digital Transformation." It is achieved when the user is able to produce and share information and knowledge with some level of innovation and creativity. This level is achieved, for example, when someone joins a virtual community, creates a blog, app, or other digital interface.

The figure below has been removed from the article. It represents the view of the authors (Fig. 3.1).

They conclude the presentation of this vision by stating that:

> Users do not necessarily follow a sequential path at each stage. They will draw upon whatever is relevant for the life-project they are currently addressing; the pattern is more one of random rather than serial access, although there will be many cases where certain low level knowledge and skill is necessary in order to develop or understand material from a higher level. (Martin & Grudziecki, 2006, p. 255)

We would like to conclude this chapter by defending the idea that "digital literacy" is a permanent process. The levels or "stages" proposed by Martin and Grudziecki (2006) are redone daily by many of us. How come?

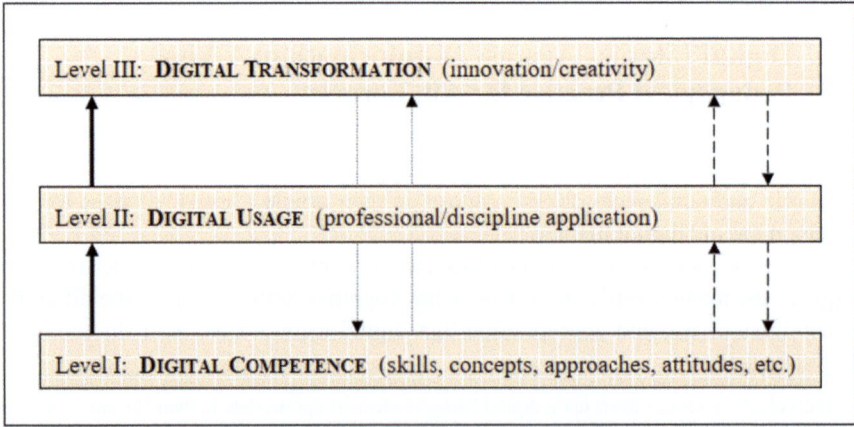

Fig. 3.1 Levels of digital literacy (Martin & Grudziecki, 2006, p. 255)

I'll describe a case. New applications or digital interfaces are often released. We are often forced to learn how to deal with them in order to fulfill some obligation or need. We cannot have a "Digital Usage" because we do not have a "Digital Competence" to deal with this novelty. One of the challenges I currently face is related to the use and appropriation of the services and facilities offered by "Já É": a digital platform of the City of Rio de Janeiro that allows citizens to request public services, point out urban problems, and follow up on requests to the municipal administration. It was created to facilitate communication between the population and the government, speeding up the resolution of issues related to infrastructure, cleaning, mobility, and other services. Once I can download this app on my phone, I still feel like someone digitally (in)competent. As a user, I don't feel like I have enough manual and cognitive skills to take advantage of this app. One detail: without it, I don't get on public transport.

A second case may be mentioned. For some time, there was ORKUT: a pioneering social network, launched in 2004. It was one of the first social networks to gain global popularity, especially in Brazil, where it became a cultural phenomenon. I even developed research that analyzed the encouragement of anorexia in young females in an Orkut community. (Ramos et al., 2011). The virtual community "Perfection is a 24-hour effort," available on ORKUT, was chosen, among others, because it was the one that had the largest number of people registered at the time of the observation (1616 participants), carried out between January and March 2009. It peaked in users between 2007 and 2011, but lost ground to Facebook. In 2014, Google decided to disable Orkut because it couldn't compete with Facebook, Instagram, and WhatsApp. The main virtual community became Facebook. I myself developed research analyzing a virtual community of chronic kidney patients on Facebook (Pereira Neto et al., 2019). The research was carried out during July 2016 in two virtual communities: "I do hemodialysis Brazil" and "Hemodialysis: a gift of life." At the opportunity, we concluded that:

> this chapter reflects on the relationship between empowerment, "expert patient," and the biomedical model by examining two online groups on Facebook that include chronic kidney patients and their relatives, friends, and caregivers. (Pereira Neto et al., 2019, p. 1)

In recent times, Facebook is no longer the main social network, being replaced by Instagram. All these changes involved millionaire sums. They forced users to go through a digital literacy process that involved levels 1 and 2, proposed by Martin and Grudziecki (2006).

If we are referring to disinformation, the examples are even more worrying. The other day, I received a message on my WhatsApp account that seemed to be from the "Brazilian Mail and Telegraph Company" (ECT). At the top of the message was the company logo. The formal text suggested that it was true information. ECT is a Brazilian federal public company responsible for the execution of the mail sending and delivery system throughout Brazil. It also distributes parcels throughout the national territory. The message had my full name and other personal and confidential data, including my home address. The message asked me to pay for a parcel to be sent to my residence. I was tempted to click on the indicated link and make the payment to receive the alleged parcel. I paused for a moment and thought to myself, "Why am I getting this message if I haven't bought anything that would be delivered through the post office?" I gave it a second thought and decided not to make the payment. The next day, I went to the post office closest to my house. When I got there, I showed the message to a clerk. She told me that it was not company policy to make such charges. Then she showed me that at the top of the billing form, there was an electronic address that did not match that of the ECT. The address was "correioparados.com". This address is fake and the information is fraudulent!

For this reason, we propose that digital literacy practices become public programs and policies to be carried out inside and outside schools. Digital literacy should be integrated into primary care activities so that the user can empower themselves with information and be able to have greater autonomy in the management of their care.

When we argue that "digital literacy" is a practice *for everyone*, we mean that it should not be restricted to those digitally excluded, as mentioned at the beginning of this chapter. I am a digitally included person, but I often face challenges posed by information and communication technologies that give testimony that I am not as literate as I thought. We mention *"forever"* because new apps and devices are offered to us on a daily basis. This seems to be an inherent trend in new information and communication technologies.

References

Ban, S., Kim, Y., & Seomun, G. (2024). Digital health literacy: A concept analysis. *Digital Health, 7*(10), 20552076241287894.

Bodie, G. D., & Dutta, M. J. (2008). Understanding health literacy for strategic health marketing: eHealth literacy, health disparities, and the digital divide. *Health Marketing Quarterly, 25*(1–2), 175–203.

Borges Do Nascimento, I. J., Pizarro, A. B., Almeida, J. M., et al. (2022). Infodemics and health misinformation: A systematic review of reviews. *Bulletin of the World Health Organization, 100*(9), 544–561.

Brazilian Network Information Center - NIC.br. (2023). *Executive summary - Survey on the use of information and communication technologies in Brazilian households - ICT Households 2022*. [online] CETIC.Br. Brazilian Internet Steering Committee - CGI.br. Accessed April 30, 2025, from https://cetic.br/media/docs/publicacoes/2/20230825143002/executive_summary_ict_households_2022.pdf

Campanozzi, L. L., Gibelli, F., Bailo, P., et al. (2023). The role of digital literacy in achieving health equity in the third millennium society: A literature review. *Frontiers in Public Health, 11*, 1109323.

Carretero Gomez, S., Vuorikari, R., & Punie, Y. (2017). *DigComp 2.1: The Digital Competence Framework for Citizens with eight proficiency levels and examples of use*. [online] JRC Publications Repository. European Commission. Accessed April 30, 2025, from https://publications.jrc.ec.europa.eu/repository/handle/JRC106281

Castells, M. (1996). *The rise of the network society*. Blackwell.

Castells, M., Fernández-Ardèvol, M., Qiu, J. L., et al. (2007). *Mobile communication and society: A global perspective*. MIT Press.

European Commission. (2022). *Guidelines for teachers and educators on tackling disinformation and promoting digital literacy through education and training*. [online] Publications Office of the European Union. European Commission. Accessed April 30, 2025, from https://op.europa.eu/en/publication-detail/-/publication/a224c235-4843-11ed-92ed-01aa75ed71a1/language-en

Eysenbach, G. (2020). How to fight an infodemic: The four pillars of infodemic management. *Journal of Medical Internet Research, 22*(6), e21820.

Feldmann, P., & Belluzzo, L. (2011). *Telecomunicações, reforma e convergência: a experiência brasileira*. Saraiva.

Fischer, C. (1992). *America calling: A social history of the telephone to 1940*. University of California Press.

Gilster, P. (1997). *Digital Literacy*. New York: John Wiley & Sons, Inc.

International Telecommunication Union. (2025). *Brazil - Individuals using the Internet*. [online] DataHub - ITU. Accessed April 30, 2025, from https://datahub.itu.int/data/?e=BRA&c=701&i=11624

Jafar, Z., Quick, J. D., Rimányi, E., et al. (2024). Social media and digital inequity: Reducing health inequities by closing the digital divide. *International Journal of Environmental Research and Public Health, 21*(11), 1420.

Martin, A., & Grudziecki, J. (2006). DigEuLit: Concepts and tools for digital literacy development. *Innovation in Teaching and Learning in Information and Computer Sciences, 5*(4), 249–267.

Mercer, D. (2006). *The telephone: The life story of a technology*. Greenwood Press.

Paige, S. R., Stellefson, M., Kriege, J. L., et al. (2018). Proposing a transactional model of eHealth literacy: Concept analysis. *Journal of Medical Internet Research, 20*(10), e10175.

Peng, D., & Yu, Z. (2022). A literature review of digital literacy over two decades. *Education Research International, 2022*(1), 2533413.

Pereira Neto, A., Lima, J. F., Barbosa, L., et al. (2019). Internet, expert patient, and empowerment: Activity profiles in virtual communities of chronic kidney patients. In A. Pereira Neto & M. Flynn (Eds.), *Internet and health in Brazil: Challenges and trends* (pp. 87–111). Springer.

Puig, B., Blanco-Anaya, P., & Pérez-Maceira, J. J. (2021). "Fake news" or real science? Critical thinking to assess information on COVID-19. *Frontiers in Education, 6*, 646909.

Ramos, J., Pereira Neto, A., & Bagrichevsky, M. (2011). Pro-anorexia cultural identity: Characteristics of a lifestyle in a virtual community. *Interface (Botucatu), 15*(37), 447–460.

Reddy, P., Sharma, B., & Chaudhary, K. (2020). Digital literacy: A review of literature. *International Journal of Technoethics (IJT), 11*(2), 65–94.

Shanahan, M., & Bahia, K. (2024). *The State of Mobile Internet Connectivity 2024*. [online] GSMA. Accessed April 30, 2025, from https://www.gsma.com/r/wp-content/uploads/2024/10/The-State-of-Mobile-Internet-Connectivity-Report-2024.pdf

Silva, E. (2022). A Transformação Digital e as Profissões do Futuro [Digital Transformation and the Professions of the Future]. *The Trends Hub, 1*(2), 1–4.

Snyder, H. (2019). Literature review as a research methodology: An overview and guidelines. *Journal of Business Research, 104*, 333–339.

Sulzer, A. (2018). (Re)conceptualizing digital literacies before and after the election of Trump. *English Teaching: Practice and Critique, 17*(2), 58–71.

Teixeira, P. M. N. (2023). Estados da Arte: aparando arestas na compreensão dessa modalidade de pesquisa [States of art: Trimming edges in the understanding of this type of research]. *Science & Education, 29*, e23034.

Temelkova, M. (2023). A concept for restructuring the production systems into cyber-physical production systems. In A. K. Nagar, D. S. Jat, D. K. Mishra, et al. (Eds.), *Intelligent sustainable systems: Selected papers of World S4 2022* (6th WorldS4 2022, London, August 2022) (Vol. 1, pp. 785–794). Springer Nature Singapore.

Tinmaz, H., Lee, Y. T., Fanea-Ivanovici, M., et al. (2022). A systematic review on digital literacy. *Smart Learning Environments, 9*, 21.

Turkle, S. (2011). *Alone together: Why we expect more from technology and less from each other*. Basic Books.

Valverde-Berrocoso, J., González-Fernández, A., & Acevedo-Borrega, J. (2025). Disinformation and multiliteracy: A systematic review of the literature. *Comunicar, 70*, 93–105.

Whittemore, R., & Knafl, K. (2005). The integrative review: Updated methodology. *Journal of Advanced Nursing, 52*(5), 546–553.

Yoon, J. (2020). *Conceptualization and assessment of digital health technology literacy.* Sungkyunkwan University.

Zhong, X., Ye, M., Zhang, D., et al. (2025). The current state of digital literacy research in China: A literature review. *Journal of Digital Pedagogy, 4*(1), 3–23.

Chapter 4
Fact-Checking: Necessary and Urgent

Abstract We live in the Information Society, under the aegis of "Post-Mass Media." Through it, many users create and share information, revealing their interests, worldviews, knowledge, and narratives that spread on social networks. This information may be incorrect and have the deliberate intention of deceiving or causing harm to the interlocutors. Fact-checking is one of the most important, structured, and widespread initiatives in the world to fight disinformation. It is carried out by independent private institutions or linked to some traditional media. There is still no common assessment method to verify the facts. In addition, the effects of this initiative are not yet evident, and its funding is uncertain. There is still resistance to accepting their verdict. However, fact-checking is necessary and urgent.

Keywords Disinformation · Health communication · Internet use · Social media

4.1 Introduction

Nowadays, many citizens create and share information, revealing their interests, worldviews, knowledge, and narratives that spread across different platforms, social networks, virtual communities, blogs, and instant news updates. This information may be incorrect and have the deliberate intention of deceiving or causing harm to the interlocutors. False information can influence public opinion, fuel political polarization, interfere with our state of health, and even incite violence. Fighting misinformation is a challenge to be faced. Fact-checking is one of the most important, structured, and widespread initiatives in the world to fight disinformation. To analyze it, it is necessary to situate it in the context in which we find ourselves: The Information Society where "Post-Mass Media" predominate.

This chapter is divided into two parts. In the first, I will describe some characteristics of the Information Society where "Post-Mass Media" play a prominent role. Next, I present some aspects of fact-checking agencies in the world, emphasizing the problem of financing these initiatives. The methods adopted in the verification of the facts, the evaluation of their impact, and the analyses that seek to explain the resistance to their verdict will also be the object of reflection.

"Mass Media" and "Post-Mass Media." André Lemos introduced these concepts 20 years ago. Lemos is one of the most important Brazilian social analysts who has been striving to understand the world we live in. His book "Cibercultura: Tecnologia e Vida Social na Cultura Contemporânea" (Cyberculture: Technology and Social Life in Contemporary Culture) was published in 2002 in Brazil (Lemos, 2002). It is the printed version of his doctoral thesis, defended in 1995 at the University of Paris in France. This book was released around the same time that Castells (1996) (*The Rise of the Network Society*), Lévy (1997) ("Cyberculture"), and Bell (2001) ("Introduction to Cybercultures") published their works. These four authors discuss in their works how digital technologies (Internet, networks, artificial intelligence) reconfigure social, economic, political, and cultural relations. In them, cyberculture is not seen only as a set of technologies, but as a way of life that redefines identities, (virtual) communities, and everyday practices.

Lemos (2002) established a conceptual distinction between "Mass Media" and "Post-Mass Media," that we consider important to remember. It helps us to put into context the construction and expansion of fact-checking agencies.

According to him, "Mass Media" are centralized and unidirectional. The production of information is controlled by large corporations and/or obeys political and/or economic interests. The information they disseminate is produced by a nucleus that sends messages to multiple receivers at the same time, such as in a "broadcasting," a communication method that allows a content-producing nucleus to send messages to multiple receivers at the same time. A structure where the few communicate to the many. In it, the public has little chance of appropriating the content, which is produced under strict editorial control. I often jokingly say in my classes that "at this moment when we are in the classroom, the newsrooms of TV news programs, which will air tonight, are deciding what we are going to know and what we are not going to know." I add that "they are also the ones who define how this information is to be disseminated." Although it seems like a joke, this phrase carries a truth. In "Mass Media," a few content producers determine the information that will (not) be disseminated, how long it will last, and what point of view they will stand for. In addition, the content is static, that is, there is little possibility of modification or reappropriation of the information by the public. The structure is vertical, as few people produce the content and determine how the information will be received and consumed by other citizens.

For Lemos (2002), "Post-Mass Media" are different as they are decentralized and interactive. In addition, production does not have a single nucleus. In this case, the information can be produced and shared by any user, as long as he is a digitally included person with the skill and dexterity to deal with different technological devices. The information in the "Post-Mass Media" would be *crowdsourced*. This term is a combination of the words *"crowd"* and *"outsourcing."* In "Post-Mass Media," communication does not have a single content-producing core. The structure is organized by the many to the many. There is an active participation of users in their content production and dissemination through social networks, blogs, and

4.1 Introduction

other collaborative platforms. Content production is open. There is a possibility of modification, sharing, and appropriation of the contents. It is a horizontal structure. In this case, there are a few barriers between producers and consumers. For this reason, they are called "*prosumers.*" This expression derives from joining the words "producer" and "consumer." It is a dream of unprecedented freedom in the creation and dissemination of information in the history of humanity.

In the introduction to the reissue of the same work, published in 2020, Lemos (2020) makes a series of caveats that relativize the dream mentioned above. According to him, reality has changed a lot. The "platformization of Society" (Van Dijck et al., 2018, p. 24), algorithms, and the increasing use of data threaten our privacy and individual freedom. The information we naively make available on digital platforms (Google, Facebook, etc.) turns into commodities, creating "surveillance capitalism" (Zuboff, 2019, p. 14). According to Lemos (2020, p. 11), the "tipping point" of cyberculture took place with the personalization of information for commercial purposes and the related induction for the consumption of specific products and services. Gradually, the Internet became a great commercial and advertising machine. Algorithms are increasingly sophisticated. They get information from users, build their profile, and offer personalized (customized) information to product, process, and service providers.

Lemos (2020) admits, however, that despite everything, the "[…] open dimension and the sharing of information and knowledge is still present today" (Lemos, 2020, p. 11).

As mentioned in the other chapters of this book, "Post-Mass Media" allows many users to create and publish information, revealing their interests, worldviews, knowledge, and narratives that spread on social networks. The large volume of information that is conveyed may be outdated, incomplete, incorrect, or with (or without) the deliberate intention to deceive or cause damage to the interlocutors.

Two initial questions are to be asked in this chapter: Is "Mass Media" the place of truth? Does it continue to dominate the information market after the emergence of "Post-Mass Media"? Let's look at the first question.

There is, in common sense, a mistaken idea that disinformation began with the advent and expansion of new information and communication technologies. For many citizens, disinformation would be an asset of the "Post-Mass Media."

In my view, disinformation is not the exclusive asset of "Post-Mass Media." "Mass Media" sometimes offer outdated, incomplete, and incorrect information with (or without) the deliberate intention of misleading interlocutors.

If we go back a little into recent Brazilian history, we will find examples in which "Mass Media" presented a version of the facts that did not correspond with the truth.

In Brazil, the murder of journalist Vladimir Herzog is well known. *Vlado*, as he was known by his friends, was born in 1937 in the city of Osijsk, in present-day Croatia. His family lived in Italy and emigrated to Brazil in 1942, when he was about 5 years old. Vladimir grew up in the city of São Paulo and acquired Brazilian nationality. He studied philosophy at the University of São Paulo (USP) and began his career as a journalist in 1959 at the newspaper O Estado de S. Paulo. Between 1963 and 1968, he worked at the *BBC*'s Brazilian Service in London. In 1968, he returned to Brazil and began working as a professor of television journalism at the School of Communications and Arts of the University of São Paulo (ECA-USP). In 1975, he became director of journalism at TV Cultura de São Paulo: a television channel linked to the Department of Culture of the State of São Paulo (Instituto Vladimir Herzog, 2024).

Between 1964 and 1982, Brazilian society lived under a Military Dictatorship. During the 1970s, this regime spared no effort to relentlessly pursue its enemies. The case of Rubens Paiva, brilliantly portrayed in the film "I'm Still Here," winner of the Oscar for Best Foreign Film (2025), illustrates this case. Rubens Paiva was a middle-class Brazilian citizen who was forcibly removed from his home. He was tortured and his body is still missing. Rubens Paiva and Vladimir Herzog were two Brazilian citizens, among the thousands of others, who were abused by the military regime. Herzog's case is related to the issue of disinformation promoted by the "Mass Media." For this reason, we will look at it in this chapter.

Herzog was found dead in one of the cells of the "Information Deployment Operations—Internal Defense Operations Center—DOI-CODI" of São Paulo on October 25, 1975. Photographer Silvaldo Leung Vieira took the picture of Vladimir Herzog dead. In the photo, we can see a man 1.82 m high hanging, with a belt tied around his neck, at a height of 1.63 m from the ground, with his feet resting on the ground, without any sign of having been suspended or of having hanged himself. However, the military version insisted, at the time, that Herzog had hanged himself. The "Mass Media" of the time replicated this version.

At the time, the two main "Mass Media" outlets in the cities of São Paulo and Rio de Janeiro published the following headlines: "Journalist hangs himself in a DOI-CODI cell" (O Estado de S. Paulo, 10/26/1975) and "Journalist kills himself in a DOI-CODI cell" (O Globo, 10/26/1975). Both reports ignored the DOI-CODI's history of violence against political prisoners. These two important "Mass Media" outlets disseminated this version, as it served the interests of the power holders who financed and supported these media outlets. These same vehicles had supported the overthrow of the constitutionally elected government and the establishment of a Military Regime. An example can be given in this regard.

I published an article in which we noted the decisive role that the newspaper Estado de São Paulo—Estadão played in the overthrow of President João Goulart, legitimately seated, and the establishment of the Military Regime in 1964 (Pereira Neto, 1999).

At the conclusion of this study, I stated that:

> The role played by *Estadão* in the decisive moment of the crisis of the Goulart Government gave this newspaper an expressive significance. When necessary, it turned Goulart into a *troublemaker*, a *threat* to Democracy [author's emphasis]. When it was the case, it demanded greater *energy* and *strong pulse* from the authorities. The Military Coup became legitimate by overthrowing a Government considered illegal. When taking power, legitimacy would be ensured by the 'revolutionary Government' and no longer by the formalism of the laws. (Pereira Neto, 1999, p. 120)

Thus, it should be noted, first of all, that "Mass Media" is not exclusively *the* place of truth of facts and information. Countless examples can be given in this regard in various parts of the world. I presented only one case that highlights the political position of important vehicles of the "Mass Media" in Brazil at a specific moment in history. In the case of Herzog's murder, we identified the spread of untruthful information. In the case of the overthrow of the legitimately elected government, analyzed in our article, "Mass Media" presents a version that meets certain interests and translates a worldview (Pereira Neto, 1999).

It should be noted, however, that this is not always the case.

Sometimes the "Mass Media" unmasks situations that only come to our knowledge through the investigation carried out by journalists working for large conglomerates of the "Mass Media." This was the case, for example, that involved Eduard Snowden, analyzed in the first chapter of this book. It is one of the most important incidents in recent history involving the unauthorized disclosure of classified US National Security Agency (NSA) documents that revealed extensive global surveillance programs. A case that brought the serious problem of invasion of privacy to the agenda. The newspapers The Guardian and The Washington Post played a decisive role in elucidating this case that occurred in 2013. In addition, every day, "Mass Media" disseminates useful and reliable information that serves to guide our daily lives and form our opinion about what is happening in our city, country, and in the world.

In any case, I believe it is important to establish some level of critical sense in relation to the media, whether they are of the Mass or Post-Mass kind.

The second question that deserves attention is the following: Does "Mass Media" continue to dominate the information market after the emergence and consolidation of "Post-Mass Media"?

In my view, at the beginning of the new millennium, the expansion and consolidation of *smartphones* definitely undermined this sovereignty. One case may illustrate this devastating trend.

Ten years ago, a colleague commented to me that her daughter, just over 20 years of age, had graduated and was going to have her own home. She wasn't getting married. She would just stop living with her mother and have her own house. She was going to live on her own in another city. As is common in Brazil, many young people, when they leave their parents' house, make a list of gifts on an Internet website for their friends and relatives to help them equip their new home. My friend's daughter's list included utensils with different values, such as plates, cutlery, stove, refrigerator, among others. The list did not include a television set. At one point, the mother asked why her daughter had not included a television set on this list. And she said, "Television for what?"

It was then that I realized that the expansion and the consolidation of "Post-Mass Media" through mobile devices were undermining the sovereignty kept until then by the "Mass Media."

To present some data attesting to this growth, I turned to the website *"Statista"* (Statista, 2024). This is an important platform that aggregates and analyzes data from more than 22,500 sources, making the information accessible to companies, researchers, and the public. Laricchia (2024) published a report in *"Statista"* stating that:

Always in our pockets or in our hands, today it is almost impossible to imagine a life without smartphones. With the introduction of Apple's iPhone in 2007, smartphones—mobile phones with more advanced computing capabilities and connectivity—revolutionized the mobile device industry. Manufacturers have quickly followed, offering consumers a wide range of smartphone brands and models. However, recent years have witnessed a stagnation of the smartphone market, with vendors trying to innovate it with new devices, including foldables and AI smartphones. (Laricchia, 2024)

Taylor (2024) published a report in *"Statista"* stating that the number of mobile *smartphone* network subscriptions worldwide rose from 3 billion 700 thousand users in 2016 to 7 billion in 2023. According to him:

> The number of smartphone mobile network subscriptions worldwide reached almost seven billion in 2023, and is forecast to exceed 7.7 billion by 2028. China, India, and the United States are the countries with the highest number of smartphone mobile network subscriptions.
> [...] The smartphone market still has high growth potential, with the smartphone penetration rate remaining lower than 70 percent in many highly populated markets, in particular China and India. (Taylor, 2024)

The above data reiterates what I had reported in previous chapters: the *smartphone* market grew at an astonishing speed! Thirty years ago, it was a luxury object, expensive, heavy, and with few features. Today, it is a lightweight, low-cost device (compared to previous models) with countless features that is used by more than half of the world's population. Its memory and speed have greatly increased. Artificial Intelligence is contributing to a new wave of innovation in these mobile devices.

In "Post-Mass Media," the user has the power to produce and share information on different platforms, at low cost, which can be accessed by thousands of citizens in the most different corners of the planet. For Wardle and Derakhshan (2017), this condition allows three types of "misinformation" to be created:

> Mis-information is when false information is shared, but no harm is meant.
> Dis-information is when false information is knowingly shared to cause harm.
> Mal-information is when genuine information is shared to cause harm, often by moving information designed to stay private into the public sphere. (Wardle & Derakhshan, 2017, p. 5)

Brennen et al. (2020), in a report published in the *Digital News Report* of the Reuters Institute and the University of Oxford, recently demonstrated that fake news is mainly found on social networks. In the same study, Brennen et al. (2020) concluded that:

> In terms of formats, most (59%) of the misinformation in our sample involves various forms of reconfiguration, where existing and often true information is spun, twisted, recontextualised, or reworked. Less misinformation (38%) was completely fabricated. [...] The reconfigured misinformation accounts for 87% of social media interactions in the sample; the fabricated content, for 12%. (Brennen et al., 2020, p. 1)

To adulterate or manufacture these contents, disinformation agents employed simple photo or video editing techniques that do not require a very sophisticated technological domain. This is possible because any citizen with expertise and

4.1 Introduction

certain specific skills in information and communication technologies can make these modifications and make this information available in the virtual environments in which they participate. In this sense, Kim et al. (2021) warn:

> Depending on the situation, people can quickly change their roles from fake news consumers to creators, or vice versa (with or without their intention). Furthermore, news creation and consumption are the most fundamental aspects that form the relationship between news and people. (Kim et al., 2021, p. 2)

It should be remembered that this information can be shared quickly among friends, followers, or even strangers in a few seconds; that is, the spread of fake news is very fast. This framework becomes even more complex, as users have increasingly sought interactive media to obtain information, abandoning "Mass Media."

According to Kim et al. (2021):

> The public's perception of news and the major media of news consumption has gradually changed. The public no longer passively consumes news exclusively through traditional news organizations with specific formats (e.g., the inverted pyramid style, verified sources) nor view those news simply as a medium for information acquisition. [...] As a result, the public began to prefer interactive media, in which new information could be acquired, their opinions can be shared, and they can discuss the news with other news consumers [...]. (Kim et al., 2021, p. 7)

In the first part of this chapter, we demonstrate that "Mass Media" fail to tell the truth. They are not *the* (only) place of truth. In it, interests, visions, and ideologies interfere with the quality of the information disseminated. We emphasize, on the other hand, that "Mass Media" have played a relevant role in serious investigations that have marked history, as in the one involving Snowden. The "Post-Mass Media" have played an equally relevant role in denouncing the atrocities committed by the police force, as was the case involving George Floyd, analyzed in the first chapter of this book. In "Post-Mass Media," some wrong information is posted with the intention of causing harm. The ease in the production and sharing of information, characteristic of "Post-Mass Media," made this problem even more serious, especially given the place that portable devices have come to occupy in contemporary times.

Given this context, fact-checking agencies have begun to be built in recent years: organizations that verify the veracity of circulating information published, above all, in the "Post-Mass Media."

We will present below some characteristics of the fact-checking agencies in the world, emphasizing the issue of financing these initiatives and the analyses that seek to explain the resistance to their verdict.

4.2 Fact-Checking in the World

Fact Check: the interest in this topic/problem is recent. Lauer and Graves (2024) admit that "The worldwide fact-checking movement has grown rapidly over the last decade and achieved remarkable prominence" (Lauer & Graves, 2024, p. 1). The growth in the number of institutions focused on fact-checking in recent years, in various parts of the world, reiterates this analysis. These organizations display a diverse range of structures and missions.

To try to bring these initiatives together under a single coordination, the "International Fact-Checking Network" (IFCN) was created in 2015 by the Poynter Institute. It presents itself as an institution that "advocates for information integrity in the global fight against misinformation and supports fact-checkers through networking, capacity building and collaboration" (DevelopmentAid, 2025).

In 2024, Stencel et al. (2024) of Duke University's Sanford School of Public Policy identified 439 fact-checking initiatives in 111 countries (Stencel et al., 2024). In 2025, 151 of these checking agencies were affiliated with IFCN, spread across 65 countries where 80 languages are spoken. Thus, approximately one-third of all existing verification agencies in the world were affiliated with IFCN in 2025. In order for a verification agency to integrate the IFCN, it must undergo an external evaluation process.

> Through this process, an organization must exhibit a commitment to nonpartisanship and fairness, transparency of sources, transparency of funding and organization, transparency of methodology, and a commitment to open and honest corrections. (International Fact-Checking Network, 2025a)

Cazzamatta (2025) made an effort to summarize and classify fact-checking initiatives into two groups: one is composed of agencies directly or indirectly affiliated with "Mass Media" ("established media companies"). They were called by Cazzamatta (2025, p. 3) "editorial fact-checkers." The other group includes initiatives that act independently, in "Non-Government Organizations," institutions of civil society, or the university environment that were called "independents" by the same author (Cazzamatta, 2025, p. 3).

We will initially look at some fact-checking initiatives linked to important "Mass Media" communication companies in different parts of the world and then offer some examples of "independent" agencies. Next, I will discuss how these initiatives survive financially. I will close this chapter by presenting some analyses that seek to explain why some citizens insist on considering some facts true even after their falsity has been proven.

In Brazil, two of the most important "Mass Media" companies sought to play the role of checking agencies. One is called "Estadão Verifica." It is under the guidance of the newspaper *Estado de São Paulo*, known as "Estadão": one of the most important, traditional, and influential organs of the "Mass Media" in Brazil. Its team is willing to analyze suspicious content that goes viral on social networks and WhatsApp. It presents itself as follows:

Estadão Verifica, created in 2018, is the fact-checking center of the newspaper *O Estado de S. Paulo*. We participate in the fight against disinformation on social networks, giving priority to content that may cause harm to individuals or groups. (Jornal O Estado de São Paulo, 2020).

"Fato ou Fake" is another Brazilian "editorial fact-checker" (Portal G1, 2025). It is linked to the most important communication and information group in the country: Sistema Globo—one of the largest media and entertainment conglomerates in Brazil and the world, with 120 million viewers per day.

Let us now look at two "editorial fact-checkers" existing in the United States of America.

The Fact Checker is linked to the Washington Post. Its subtitle mentions "The truth behind the rhetoric" (The Washington Post, 2025). In this case, the reading of the checked information is only allowed to subscribers of this newspaper. The other North American verification site is "AP Fact Check," linked to the "Associated Press." It states that the user will: "Verify the latest news with 'AP Fact Check'. AP fact checkers fight misinformation by debunking false and misleading claims" (The Associated Press, 2025a). As soon as the website is accessed, this advertisement appears: "Support a free and independent press. The AP remains steadfast in its mission to inform the world with accurate, factual, and nonpartisan news—as it has for nearly 180 years" (The Associated Press, 2025a). "Your donation will help The Associated Press continue its mission to advance the power of fact-based journalism" (The Associated Press, 2025b).

In Europe, Agence France-Presse stands out in France. It is one of the largest fact-checking organizations, with teams located in dozens of offices around the world. Its website states that its mission "is to provide accurate, balanced and impartial coverage of news wherever and whenever it happens in the world on a continuous basis" (Agence France-Presse, 2023).

The presence of "Mass Media" in fact-checking may be related to the fact that these media outlets intend to position themselves in defense of the truth of the facts. This repositioning may be related to the credibility crisis experienced by the "Mass Media" in the world. Recent data corroborate this idea.

The "Reuters Institute for the Study of Journalism" publishes annually since 2012, the *Digital News Report*. Its objective has been to obtain data that allows analyses to be made regarding the evolution of public opinion on media trust, misinformation, platform changes, and news consumption habits. For the preparation of the last edition, launched in 2024 (Newman et al., 2024), 2000 questionnaires were applied in each of the 47 participating countries on six continents. Among the conclusions available, there is this one:

> Generally, younger people, people with low income, and people with lower levels of formal education tend to trust the news less. These are also groups that are often less well served by the news media, and generally less likely to think that the media cover people like them fairly, as we showed in our 2021 Digital News Report. (Newman et al., 2024, p. 34)

As we have just observed, part of the "Mass Media" has built instances aimed at verifying the facts. This initiative itself is worthy of praise. The communication environment is contaminated by misinformation. Ideally, we should have a greater number of "editorial fact-checkers" interested in unraveling the facts independently and transparently.

I will present below the performance of some "independent" agencies in the world, focused on fact-checking.

In the United States of America, "*FactCheck.org*" stands out: a project of the "Annenberg Public Policy Center" of the University of Pennsylvania. It is stated on its website that:

> We are a nonpartisan, nonprofit 'consumer advocate' for voters who aims to reduce the level of deception and confusion in U.S. politics. [...] Our goal is to apply the best practices of both journalism and scholarship, and to increase public knowledge and understanding. (FactCheck.org, 2025)

In Germany, we can mention "*Corretiv.*" They understand that:

> *Correctiv* is a public interest media company that strengthens democracy. With a multi-award winning editorial team, we champion investigative journalism. We stimulate public debates, collaborate with citizens in our research and promote society with our educational programs. (Correctiv, 2025)

In the United Kingdom, "Full Fact" *stands* out. When opening their website, there is a very objective warning stating that: "Follow Full Fact to stay informed, challenge falsehoods, and stand up for accuracy" (Full Fact, 2024). It declares its mission as follows:

> Our mission is to create a better information environment to improve trust. We're determined to help people determine what's based on fact rather than fiction, avoid the real-life harms that flow from being duped or scammed and be active democratic citizens. It's about enabling them to make informed choices on the issues that matter to them. (Full Fact, 2025)

Thus, if we compare the initiatives linked to "Mass Media" with those called "independent," we could say that the former benefit from the infrastructure, financing, and broader reach of their media parent companies, although they come across editorial restrictions. Meanwhile, "independents" enjoy greater editorial freedom, but often face financial problems and have a smaller reach (Cazzamatta, 2025).

What are the methods these agencies use to fact-check?

4.3 Fact-Checking Methods

The "International Fact-Checking Network" presents on its website the "IFCS Code of Principles." Below is a brief presentation and analysis of the five principles it contains.

The first recommends that "signatory institutions" do not take into account the party, political, or ideological affiliation of the person responsible for issuing the information when making the verification ("A commitment to Non-partisanship and Fairness"). At a certain point in the text, it states that:

4.3 Fact-Checking Methods

> Signatory organizations fact-check claims using the same standard for every fact check. They do not concentrate their fact-checking on any one side. They follow the same process for every fact check and let the evidence dictate the conclusions. Signatories do not advocate or take policy positions on the issues they fact-check. (International Fact-Checking Network, 2025b)

For the "International Fact-Checking Network," this stance can prevent the verification carried out from being influenced by the political position of the evaluator.

The second principle suggests that the results of the checks are accompanied by the respective sources used by the "signatory institutions" when carrying out the verification ("A commitment to Standards and Transparency of Sources"). It states that:

> Signatories want their readers to be able to verify findings themselves. Signatories provide all sources in sufficient detail that readers can replicate their work, except in cases where a source's personal security could be compromised. In such cases, signatories provide as much detail as possible. (International Fact-Checking Network, 2025b)

The third proposes that the "signatory institutions" responsible for the verification make public the institutions that financed the activity ("A Commitment to Transparency of Funding & Organization"). It states that:

> Signatory organizations are transparent about their funding sources. If they accept funding from other organizations, they ensure that funders have no influence over the conclusions the fact-checkers reach in their reports. Signatory organizations detail the professional background of all key figures in the organization and explain the organizational structure and legal status. (International Fact-Checking Network, 2025b)

The fourth principle recommends that the verification method used ("A Commitment to Standards and Transparency of Methodology") be clear and understandable. Users need to know how the verifiers performed their work. It states that: "Signatories explain the methodology they use to select, research, write, edit, publish and correct their fact checks. They encourage readers to send claims to fact-check and are transparent on why and how they fact-check" (International Fact-Checking Network, 2025b).

The fifth criterion proposes that those responsible for checking carry out their work openly ("A Commitment to an Open & Honest Corrections Policy"). It states that:

> Signatories publish their corrections policy and follow it scrupulously. They correct clearly and transparently in line with the corrections policy, seeking so far as possible to ensure that readers see the corrected version. (International Fact-Checking Network, 2025b)

The International Fact-Checking Network understands that a verification agency's verdict is more likely to be accepted if it complies with the IFCS Code of Principles. These principles have been adopted by different verification agencies around the world.

One of the examples in this regard was observed by Moreno-Gil and Salgado-de Dios (2023). They assessed whether the four Spanish fact-checking platforms followed the "IFCS Code of Principles." They concluded that:

This qualitative approach offers new and significant evidence of how the main Spanish fact-checking platforms are achieving most of the accountability principles established by the IFCN, especially in the implementation of a standard methodology within the verification process. (Moreno-Gil & Salgado-de Dios, 2023, p. 294)

The "IFCs Code of Principles" is not a consensus.

Vinhas and Bastos (2025) criticized the way in which the IFCN proposes that fact-checks be carried out. According to Vinhas and Bastos (2025), these principles can be valid in the "Western, Educated, Industrialized, Rich, and Democratic countries" (WEIRD). However, they are not appropriate in countries in the Southern Hemisphere, such as poor countries where authoritarian regimes that curtail freedom of expression predominate. In addition, according to them, the IFCN principles emphasize behavioral problems, stating that:

We review these findings against the literature in the area and argue that the prevailing framework of fact-checking, where misinformation and disinformation are reduced to individual and behavioral problems, underplays the social and historical dimensions driving disinformation and propaganda. (Vinhas & Bastos, 2025, p. 256)

For Vinhas and Bastos (2025), this perspective minimizes the social and historical dimensions that drive disinformation and propaganda. For them, a fact check should be carried out that takes into account the political and cultural tension in which the facts are built.

The set of strategies devised by non-WEIRD fact-checking organizations also call for a renewed understanding of how mis- and disinformation manifests socially, as their work consistently extends beyond gauging the accuracy of individual information and promoting factual reasoning. (Vinhas & Bastos, 2025, p. 257)

Vinhas and Bastos (2025) conducted a study verifying whether the same IFCN verification tool, adopted in countries that are Western, Educated, Industrialized, Rich, and Democratic (WEIRD), can be applied outside this context. Thirty-seven fact-checking experts from 35 organizations in 27 countries in Africa, Asia, Latin America, and Eastern Europe were interviewed. Vinhas and Bastos (2025) concluded that disinformation is a context-driven social malady. It is not a behavioral problem that needs to be corrected.

Our findings emphasize the contextual nature of the falsehoods that these professionals deal with on a daily basis, and the many strategies they employ to navigate cultural and political obstacles while strengthening social cohesion locally. (Vinhas & Bastos, 2025, p. 256)

In my view, the performance of fact-checking agencies may vary from one context to another. This is because some verification agencies suffer, in their respective countries, hostility, opposition, and even persecution of their performance, especially in countries where press freedom hardly exists. This is the case, above all, of countries that are located outside the territorial limits of the WEIRD.

The "V-Dem Institute" belongs to the Department of Political Science at the University of Gothenburg, Sweden. It has the largest database on democracy in the world, with more than 30 million data points for 202 countries between 1789 and 2021. More than 3700 researchers and other experts in different countries linked to the Institute measure hundreds of different indicators of democracy. The report published in 2025 (Nord et al., 2025) concluded that "70 per cent of the world's population now live in dictatorships" (University of Gothenburg, 2022). The debate about the methods and criteria for fact-checking does not stop here.

Cazzamatta (2025) conducted a literature review in 3154 articles that analyzed the experience of fact-checking of 23 organizations in 8 countries in Europe and Latin America. She identified 17 distinct debunking techniques through inductive and deductive approaches.

Cazzamatta (2025) concludes her study by stating that:

> Although several studies suggest that organizations are becoming more similar in their practices and methods as they move toward institutionalization [...], this paper reveals that significant variation in verification strategies persists at a deeper level. (Cazzamatta, 2025, p. 18–19)

Thus, the principles of verification of facts proposed by the IFCN have been the subject of reflection and criticism by several authors. There is no internationally established consensus on how this verification should be carried out. The debate on fact-checking methods seems to be open.

What about funding? How do these checking agencies survive economically?

4.4 The Financing of Fact-Checking Agencies

Data from Duke Reporter's Lab show that the vast majority of initiatives in the United States and Western Europe remain tied to traditional news outlets, while most fact-checkers in Africa, Asia, Latin America, and Eastern Europe operate as independent organizations (Stencel et al., 2022).

The problem of financing fact-checking initiatives is very important, as the act of financing can interfere with the trustworthiness of the verification.

When browsing the page of the English checking agency "Full Fact," I found a list of contributing institutions and citizens that contains 27 institutions and the respective amounts they donated (Full Fact, 2023). In this list, it appears that, in 2023, Google contributed 522,000 pounds and Meta more than 370,000 pounds, as part of the "Third Party Fact-Checking Program."

I did a similar investigation into the other "independent" initiatives and found that one of the checking agencies in Brazil, called "*Aos Fatos*," had received similar financial support.

This checking agency started operating in 2015. It presents itself as having been created "with technical resources and own investment of its creators." It appears that:

> 'Aos Fatos' is a journalistic organization dedicated to combating disinformation, covering technopolitics and checking facts. [...] it combines technology and journalistic investigation to inform about the lies that the powerful tell, endorse and finance. (Aos Fatos, 2025)

However, it announces on its website that:

[...] has been part of Meta's 3PFC (*Third Party Fact-Checking Program*) project since 2018, through which it licenses verifications of potentially misleading content circulating on Facebook, Instagram and WhatsApp platforms. (Aos Fatos, 2025)

In Europe, I identified a similar phenomenon in France's "AFP Fact Check." It presents itself as a multilingual and multicultural news agency whose mission is to provide accurate, balanced, and unbiased coverage of news wherever and whenever it happens in the world on an ongoing basis. Based on the 1957 company statute, it guarantees to act independently of the French Government, which offers support and "other influences." When this article was written, it was stated on its website that AFP had a commercial agreement with Meta 3PFC.

But what is the "Third Party Fact-Checking Program"? It is a Meta program that aims to finance fact-checking agencies.

According to Cazzamatta (2025), this program, launched in 2016 by Zuckerberg, aimed to combat the spread of disinformation and financially support fact-checkers. Without clarifying exactly the reasons for its creation, Cazzamatta (2025) admits that it occurred "in response to social and political pressures" (Cazzamatta, 2025, p. 3).

What "social and political pressures" would these be? Let's take a closer look at this question.

In 2018, Zuckerberg established partnerships with "independent" agencies linked to the "Mass Media" of fact-checking through the "Meta's Third-Party Fact-Checking Program," including the agency "Aos Fatos" in Brazil, "Full Fact" in Britain, and "AFP Fact Check" in France, mentioned above. In the same year that he made these grants, Zuckerberg was combing through the data of thousands of citizens through the scandal that later came to be known as "Cambridge Analytica." And what is that?

Hinds et al. (2020) described this scandal as follows:

In March 2018, news of the Facebook-Cambridge Analytica scandal made headlines around the world. By inappropriately collecting data from approximately 87 million users' Facebook profiles, the data analytics company, Cambridge Analytica, created psychographically tailored advertisements that allegedly aimed to influence people's voting preferences in the 2016 US presidential election. (Hinds et al., 2020, p. 1)

In 2018, The Guardian and The New York Times published reports based on interviews with a former Cambridge Analytica employee. At the time, the deponent revealed that this company obtained data from millions of users illegally and without their authorization. Thus, it was able to influence the opinion of voters in several countries during election campaigns.

Mark Zuckerberg was questioned in the United States Congress in April 2018 and in the European Parliament in May of the same year. This case was judged by the Federal Trade Commission, which, in the end, established the largest fine for invasion of privacy: US$5 billion, applied on July 24, 2019 (Federal Trade Commission, 2019). This scandal has increased debates about social media regulation, misinformation, privacy, and data protection.

4.4 The Financing of Fact-Checking Agencies

What is the relationship between the "Cambridge Analytica" scandal and the "Third-Party Fact-Checking Program"? Why did Zuckerberg decide to fund the fact-checking activities of some "independent" agencies? For Cazzamatta (2025), this initiative took place "in response to social and political pressures" (Cazzamatta, 2025, p. 3). Another plausible explanation would be related to his intention that Zuckerberg had to reposition his public image. With this financial support, he could be seen as someone who values the truth of the facts. With the "Third-Party Fact-Checking Program," Meta seeks to clean up its image after disinformation scandals arising from the lawsuit that involved "Cambridge Analytica" and avoid fines, laws, and government control.

Zuckerberg's strategy was not restricted to the "Full Fact," "Aos Fatos," or the "AFP Fact Check." Continuing the investigation, I found that the budget of the "Third-Party Fact-Checking Program" also had a broader address: the *International Fact-Checking Network*.

At the end of 2022, IFCN received a $12 million grant from Meta (Lauer & Graves, 2024). Affiliated agencies should submit projects to obtain this support. In 2023, the *International Fact-Checking Network* received external investment and supported 75 fact-checking projects in 47 countries. In 2024, the same association again announced the opening of funding to support fact-checking initiatives around the world. All these initiatives had the financial support of Meta. The IFCN published in April 2024 on its front page the following headline:

> $12 million Global Fact Check Fund opens applications for second year of grants.
> A partnership between Poynter's International Fact-Checking Network and Google and YouTube continues to support fact-checking initiatives worldwide. (International Fact-Checking Network, 2024)

After careful selection, this amount would be distributed among 40 fact-checking verification agencies, among the 150 that were part of the IFCN.

"Independent" vetting initiatives represent a valid and commendable civil society response to disinformation. The support that the International Fact-Checking Network has received from Meta does not deny the importance of its activities. The "International Fact-Checking Network" presents itself as an initiative that works to identify, finance, and launch proposals that address the global threat of disinformation. However, the presence of Meta as a funding institution suggests that the financial survival of the verification agencies is not an easy or safe task. This support, so it seems, has come to an end. A change that coincides with the election of Donald Trump as President of the United States of America.

In April 2025, Angie Holan, Director of the International Fact-Checking Network, made the following public announcement:

> Two heavy blows hit fact-checking in 2025. In January, Meta's Mark Zuckerberg announced his decision to end its third-party fact-checking in the United States. The program paid fact-checkers to help Meta identify and flag hoaxes and other false information on its platform; the program's end means less money for fact-checkers and less distribution via one of the world's largest social media companies. Right now, only U.S. fact-checkers will be affected, but it may end up being rolled out to the rest of the world in 2026. (Holan, 2025)

The second of the "heavy blows hitting fact-checking" was related to the fact that US President Donald Trump closed the United States Agency for International Development (USAID). USAID had been supporting some fact-checking initiatives because it believed it would strengthen democracy and encourage public debate.

Holan (2025) presents a solution stating that "we must make fact-checking vital to people's daily lives, reaching beyond traditional audiences." She concludes her presentation by admitting that "it's not clear what the next few years will bring" Holan, 2025). The survival of the checking agencies seems to be compromised.

Thus, there are fact-checking agencies in the four corners of the planet. However, there is still no consensus among institutions and scholars on the methods and criteria to be used in this check. In addition, financing is a great challenge to be faced.

One last question deserves to be discussed: Why do some citizens continue to accept certain fake news as true, even after it is denied?

4.5 Last Question

A case that occurred in Brazil recently may serve as a basis for this reflection. Let's see:

On September 25, 2018, an unidentified citizen posted a 44-s-long video on Facebook that features a bottle with a nipple shaped like a human penis. He informs that this bottle had been distributed by the "Workers' Party" (PT) in public daycare centers in Brazil, by the then Minister of Education, Fernando Haddad (2005/2012). The "Partido dos Trabalhadores" (PT) is a Brazilian center-left political party. In 2018, it had launched the candidacy of the former minister Fernando Haddad for the Presidency of the Republic in opposition to Bolsonaro, a candidate of the far right. According to the post, the PT's goal would be to end homophobia. The original Facebook post of the video had 2.4 million views and 71,000 shares between September 25 and 27, 2018. Bolsonaro emerged victorious with 55% of the vote.

A clarification is required.

In Brazil, voting is direct, secret, and universal (all Brazilians, over 16 years of age, have the right to vote in all elective positions). The candidate for a majority position (President, State Governor, and Mayor) is only elected if he/she obtains more than 50% of the valid votes. Thus, a second ballot is often held with the two most voted candidates of the first ballot. The first vote for President of the Republic was held on October 7: Bolsonaro obtained 46% of the votes and Haddad 29%. In the second ballot, held on October 28, Bolsonaro won 55% of the vote and Haddad 44.8%. Thus, he became the new President of the Republic of Brazil (Tribunal Superior Eleitoral, 2018).

An IDEA Big Data/Avaaz survey, conducted after the election, revealed that 83.7% of Bolsonaro voters (PSL) believed the information that the former Minister of Education—Fernando Haddad (PT)—distributed the so-called *gay kit* to children in schools. The same survey also found that 10% of Haddad voters believed this *post* to be true (Congresso em Foco, 2018).

4.5 Last Question

In the moving image, we can see only one hand holding a bottle that is accompanied by a pronouncement that tells the user the following:

> Take a look here... those of you vote for PT. This is a milk bottle distributed at the daycare center distributed for your child with the excuse of fighting homophobia. Look at the beak as it is! [that is the moment when they show the image of a penis-shaped bottle nipple]. This is what the PT and Haddad preach! Your child at five, six years of age, will drink from this bottle here (at this point it shows the image of a penis-shaped bottle nipple again). You have to vote for Bolsonaro, boy! The only way to make our children be either boys or girls. [...] This is part of the *gay kit*. (Representação no 0601530-54.2018.6.00.0000 [2018])

The *gay kit* was a pejorative designation used by the far right to refer to the set of measures included in the government program "Brazil without Homophobia," started in 2005.

Two days after the release of the video (September 27), presidential candidate Fernando Haddad denied this news. On the same day, the e-farsas fact-checking agency made the same denial, stating that:

> [...] The video, despite having had some success on social media, shows no proof that this story is real. The man speaking does not say where he would have picked up the bottle, in which school or in which daycare center. It is all very vague and lacking evidence [...]. (Lopes, 2018)

On September 28, the fact-checking agency "Aos Fatos" also denied this news, stating:

> Although several users understood the publication as satire, mocked the *post* and questioned the authenticity of the content in the comments session, there were those who expressed outrage and revolt, relying on the author's information. (Aos Fatos, 2018).

On September 28, the fact-checking agency "COMPROVA" also denied this news, stating:

> *Comprova* searched for the description of the object on Google and found that the product exists and is marketed to the adult public in *sex shops*. One of the stores that advertises the sale on the internet informed *Comprova* that the merchandise is imported. (Projeto Comprova, 2018)

The fake news continued to circulate in other montages with different photos of similar bottles, disseminated on WhatsApp in mass shots to the country's phone numbers (Traumann, 2020).

In this case, we ask: Why did some citizens continue to believe that the PT distributed a bottle like this in daycare centers in Brazil when Haddad was Minister of Education, even after this version was debunked?

Some authors have sought to explain the reasons that lead certain citizens to resist the verdict of fact-checking.

The reading and analysis of some academic articles allow us to list some possible explanations for this resistance.

A first set of authors mentions precarious information literacy as an element that hinders the acceptance of a debunking made by a fact-checking agency.

Jones-Jang et al. (2019) are some of the authors who highlight how precarious information literacy can explain the greater or lesser adherence to information that debunks fake news. The objective of the authors was:

> empirically investigates such assumptions by assessing whether individuals with greater literacy (media, information, news, and digital literacies) are better at recognizing fake news, and which of these literacies are most relevant. (Jones-Jang et al., 2019, p. 1)

The results of the investigation they carried out:

> [...] showed that information literacy, which emphasizes users' abilities to navigate and locate verified and reliable information, was positively associated with fake news identification, but the other types of literacies did not show a significant relationship. (Jones-Jang et al., 2019, p. 11)

Users who refused to admit the posting of bottles as fake may not have the mentioned skills.

A second possible explanation brings together authors who associate this resistance with the "illusory truth effect." This idea stems from a long tradition of work in cognitive science that demonstrates that prior exposure to a statement increases the likelihood that it will be considered correct by users, even if it is confirmed to be false (Udry & Barber, 2024). Repetitions also fulfill this role. In this sense, the authors state that:

> Repetition increases belief in information, a phenomenon known as the illusory truth effect. [...] Repetition even increases belief in claims that are implausible or that contradict prior knowledge. Repetition also has broader impacts beyond belief, such as increasing sharing intentions of news headlines and decreasing how unethical an act is perceived to be. (Udry & Barber, 2024, p. 1)

"The illusory truth effect" (Udry & Barber, 2024, p. 1). This may be one of the explanations that justify the fact that many citizens resist admitting that the information about the distribution of these bottles in daycare centers is false. The acceptance of this lie as truth may be associated with the fact that this false version has been repeated countless times.

For a third group of authors, psychological factors would explain why some individuals would be more likely to believe fake news, even after it had been proven wrong. "Emotional Intelligence" would be one of the variables in this sense: a relatively recent concept that seeks to integrate the intersection between emotion and cognition.

Pennycook and Rand (2018) sought to assess whether citizens who have high levels of "emotional intelligence" (EQ) are better able to assess the veracity of information than others who do not have this ability. The authors used in their investigation the "Cognitive Reflection Test" (CRT): a short psychological assessment that aims to measure analytical thinking. It assesses the extent to which the evaluated user adopts logical and deliberate reasoning in their responses. They concluded that citizens who accept fake news as truth are the same ones who had low CRT scores. They concluded that:

4.5 Last Question

> We find that CRT performance is negatively correlated with the perceived accuracy of fake news, and positively correlated with the ability to discern fake news from real news—even for headlines that align with individuals' political ideology. (Pennycook & Rand, 2018, p. 1)

In our view, the lack of "Emotional Intelligence" is even more likely in contexts laden with anxiety, anger, and/or admiration, like the one that preceded the 2018 presidential election in Brazil, ideologically polarized and loaded with different emotional appeals. In this regard, Martel et al. (2020) concluded that:

> We found that across a wide range of specific emotions, heightened emotionality at the outset of the study was predictive of greater belief in fake (but not real) news posts. […] We found both correlational and causal evidence that reliance on emotion increases belief in fake news: self-reported use of emotion was positively associated with belief in fake (but not real) news, and inducing reliance on emotion resulted in greater belief in fake (but not real) news stories compared to a control or to inducing reliance on reason. These results shed light on the unique role that emotional processing may play in susceptibility to fake news. (Martel et al., 2020, p. 1).

Ferreira (2019) observed the use of disinformation in the 2018 campaign and pointed out that the false narrative of the *gay kit* was one of the 20 most shared false narratives on social networks during the electoral period. According to the author, false content on the subject associated with children's sexuality was used on digital social networks mainly against Fernando Haddad.

It should be noted, however, that the explanations mentioned above are not the only justifications suggested by the broad specialized literature on the subject.

The last one deserves our attention. This is the one associated with the idea of "confirmation bias" and "echo chambers." "Confirmation bias" occurs when an individual seeks out and uses information to support ideas or beliefs previously held. This means that information that does not agree with his ideas or beliefs is not considered by him. By using "confirmation bias," individuals select parts of the information that confirm their previous concepts, information, and knowledge and despise others (Nickerson, 1998).

"Confirmation bias" is closely associated with "echo chambers." An "echo chamber" is an environment in which users' opinion, political learning, or beliefs are reinforced by repeated interactions with peers or similar sources. Opinions, learnings, and beliefs result from selective exposure to opinions conveyed by citizens with the same interests and values. The influence of "echo chambers" includes the exclusion of alternative perspectives. Political, administrative, and social deadlock in many contexts has been termed "*Social media induced* polarisation" (SMIP).

Modgil et al. (2024) carried out an investigation seeking to establish a relationship between SMIP and "confirmation bias" and "echo chambers." In conclusion, they stated that:

> […] The findings demonstrate that there is a reciprocal, reinforcing relationship between confirmation bias and echo chambers that accelerates SMIP, as opposed to just the social media platforms itself. Concluding, this study advances understanding of the architecture of confirmation bias that leads to echo chambers, not just in the context of global pandemics, but also in national and international events that can have devastating effects on societies. (Modgil et al., 2024, p. 431)

To some extent, this bottle became real. Reality and fiction are very close. Sometimes reality completes fiction. Sometimes fiction completes reality. In *Six Walks in the Woods of Fiction* (Eco, 1994), Umberto Eco brings together six essays derived from his lectures at Harvard University. He starts from the metaphor of the forest as a narrative labyrinth and analyzes how readers voluntarily get lost in fictional universes, seduced by the complexity of texts. The author discusses the construction of possible worlds and believable characters, highlighting how fiction creates alternative realities that demand the voluntary suspension of disbelief by the public. Bolsonaro's followers made a fictional construction true. This is another possible explanation for the resistance to fact-checking.

In any case, citing Preston et al. (2021), "Research on how to combat the false acceptance of fake news is still in its infancy." (Preston et al., 2021, p. 1).

4.6 Final Considerations

The origin of information disorder has been analyzed in this chapter. It is related to the characteristics of "Post-Mass Media" that allow many citizens to be able to create and share information, revealing their interests, worldviews, knowledge, and narratives that spread on social networks, like a virus. This information may be incorrect and have the deliberate intention of deceiving or causing harm to the interlocutors. We also analyzed the devastating consequences that disinformation has on politics and health. Fact-checking is an alternative to face this problem that today can be identified in different parts of the world.

In this sense, I echo the words of Lauer (2024) when he admits that the policy of fact-checking agencies in the world comprises similar practices that obey different rationalities.

> While united by very similar verification practices, the community of fact-checkers is remarkably diverse. Reflecting the media-political landscapes they navigate, these initiatives bring together a spectrum of professional expertise, visions, and strategies. (Lauer, 2024, p. 1)

In this chapter, it was demonstrated that there is no consensus on what methods and criteria should be used to perform this check. There are still many doubts regarding why successful information debunking fails to be believed. This is a recent social phenomenon. By the time the reader is reading this chapter, further assessments of the effects of the check will have been made. Other initiatives will have been undertaken. Other methods will have been applied. Efforts to improve fact-checking are ongoing.

The problem of the financing of "Fact-checking" leads me to another question: Should the government take on the responsibility of fact-checking? As I see it, yes. The government has an obligation to care about the health of the population. Wrong information, with or without the intention of causing harm, is harmful to health. The recent case of the infodemic that contaminated the world during the COVID-19 pandemic can serve as an example.

The study by Rocha et al. (2021) offers elements for this reflection. According to them:

> as the new coronavirus disease propagated around the world, the rapid spread of news caused uncertainty in the population. False news has taken over social media, becoming part of life for many people. (Rocha et al., 2021, p. 1)

From this finding, the authors conducted a systematic review and concluded that:

> Social-media platforms have contributed to the spread of false news and conspiracy theories during the new coronavirus pandemic. When analyzing the phenomenon of fake news in health, it is possible to observe that infodemic knowledge is part of people's lives around the world, causing distrust in Governments, researchers, and health professionals, which can directly impact people's lives and health. (Rocha et al., 2021, p. 8)

Coping with disinformation is one of the main contemporary challenges. It is eroding social understanding and democratic values. It affects different areas. Disinformation in health can lead citizens to abandon treatment, not get vaccinated, or self-medicate incorrectly, as in the case of COVID-19. It can also overcrowd hospital emergency wards, sow panic and anxiety, and contribute to disbelief in science.

The Lancet editorial, published in January 2025, admits that health misinformation, whether involuntary or deliberate, was intensified during the COVID-19 pandemic. During the pandemic, it generated anxiety and facilitated the spread of inadequate treatments that led to the death of thousands of people. In his words:

> Health misinformation (false or misleading data shared unintentionally) and disinformation (deliberately deceptive information) are not new, but the COVID-19 pandemic marked a turning point. [...] Disinformation has become a deliberate instrument to attack and discredit scientists and health professionals for political gains. The effects are destructive and damaging to public health. (The Lancet, 2025, p. 173)

In its conclusion, the editorial states that:

> Misinformation and disinformation can no longer be viewed simply as an academic nuisance, but rather they are a societal threat. Only if we recognize that threat and act proportionately can we respond to the danger and combat the tide of misinformation and disinformation that has the potential to seriously undermine public health. (The Lancet, 2025, p. 173)

We are in the midst of this informational disorder, where every day that passes, fact-checking becomes not only necessary but urgent.

References

Agence France-Press. (2023). *About AFP*. [online] Fact Check. Accessed May 7, 2025, from https://factcheck.afp.com/about-afp

Aos Fatos. (2018). *'Mamadeiras eróticas' não foram distribuídas em creches pelo PT*. [online] Aos Fatos. Accessed May 7, 2025, from https://www.aosfatos.org/noticias/mamadeiras-eroticas-nao-foram-distribuidas-em-creches-pelo-pt/

Aos Fatos. (2025). *Sobre o Aos Fatos*. [online] Aos Fatos. Accessed May 9, 2025, from https://www.aosfatos.org/sobre-o-aos-fatos/

Bell, D. (2001). *An introduction to cybercultures*. Routledge.

Brennen, J. S., Simon, F. M., Philip, R. K., et al. (2020). *Types, sources, and claims of COVID-19 misinformation*. Reuters Institute for the Study of Journalism.

Castells, M. (1996). *The rise of the network society*. Blackwell.

Cazzamatta, R. (2025). Decoding correction strategies: How fact-checkers uncover falsehoods across countries. *Journalism Studies*, 1–23.

Congresso em Foco. (2018). *Pesquisa mostra que 84% dos eleitores de Bolsonaro acreditam no kit gay*. [online] Congresso em Foco. Accessed May 7, 2025, from https://www.congressoemfoco.com.br/noticia/33044/pesquisa-mostra-que-84-dos-eleitores-de-bolsonaro-acreditam-no-kit-gay

Correctiv. (2025). *Über CORRECTIV*. [online] CORRECTIV. Accessed May 7, 2025, from https://correctiv.org/ueber-uns/

DevelopmentAid. (2025). *International Fact-Checking Network*. [online] DevelopmentAid. Accessed May 9, 2025, from https://www.developmentaid.org/donors/view/183645/international-fact-checking-network

Eco, U. (1994). *Seis passeios pelos bosques da ficção*. Companhia das Letras.

FactCheck.org. (2025). *Our Mission*. [online] FactCheck.org. Accessed May 7, 2025, from https://www.factcheck.org/about/our-mission/

Federal Trade Commission. (2019). *FTC imposes $5 billion penalty and sweeping new privacy restrictions on Facebook*. [online] Federal Trade Commission. Accessed May 7, 2025, from https://www.ftc.gov/news-events/news/press-releases/2019/07/ftc-imposes-5-billion-penalty-sweeping-new-privacy-restrictions-facebook

Ferreira, R. (2019). *Desinformação em processos eleitorais: um estudo de caso da eleição brasileira de 2018*. University of Coimbra, Coimbra [Masther's thesis]. Accessed May 7, 2025, from https://estudogeral.uc.pt/handle/10316/93397

Full Fact. (2023). *Funding - Full Fact*. [online] Full Fact. Accessed May 7, 2025, from https://fullfact.org/about/funding/

Full Fact. (2024). *Home*. [online] Full Fact. Accessed May 7, 2025, from https://fullfact.org/

Full Fact. (2025). *#FactsMatter. Here's why*. [online] Full Fact. https://fullfact.org/blog/2025/mar/facts-matter/

Hinds, J., Williams, E. J., & Joinson, A. N. (2020). "It wouldn't happen to me": Privacy concerns and perspectives following the Cambridge Analytica scandal. *International Journal of Human-Computer Studies, 143*, 102498.

Holan, A. D. (2025). *Will the future of fact-checking flourish or founder? 2025 marks a new turning point - Poynter*. [online] Poynter. Accessed May 7, 2025, from https://www.poynter.org/fact-checking/2025/angie-drobnic-holan-international-fact-checking-day/

Instituto Vladimir Herzog. (2024). *O Caso Herzog*. [online] Instituto Vladimir Herzog. Accessed May 7, 2025, from https://vladimirherzog.org/casoherzog/

International Fact-Checking Network. (2024). *International fact-checking network*. [online] Poynter. Accessed May 7, 2025, from https://www.poynter.org/ifcn/2024/12-million-global-fact-check-fund-opens-applications-for-second-year-of-grants-google-youtube/

International Fact-Checking Network. (2025a). *IFCN Code of Principles - Signatories*. [online] International Fact-Checking Network. https://ifcncodeofprinciples.poynter.org/signatories

International Fact-Checking Network. (2025b). *The commitments of the Code of Principles*. [online] International Fact-Checking Network. https://ifcncodeofprinciples.poynter.org/the-commitments

Jones-Jang, S. M., Mortensen, T., & Liu, J. (2019). Does media literacy help identification of fake news? Information literacy helps, but other literacies don't. *American Behavioral Scientist, 65*(2), 371–388.

References

Jornal O Estado de São Paulo. (2020). *Sobre o Estadão Verifica*. [online] Estadão. Accessed May 8, 2025, from https://www.estadao.com.br/estadao-verifica/recebeu-algum-boato-envie-para-checagem-do-estadao-estadao-verifica/

Kim, B., Xiong, A., Lee, D., et al. (2021). A systematic review on fake news research through the lens of news creation and consumption: Research efforts, challenges, and future directions. *PLoS One, 16*(12), e0260080.

Laricchia, F. (2024). *Smartphones - statistics & facts*. [online] Statista. Accessed May 7, 2025, from https://www.statista.com/topics/840/smartphones/#editorsPicks

Lauer, L. (2024). *Similar practice, different rationales. Political fact-checking around the world*. Springer VS.

Lauer, L., & Graves, L. (2024). How to grow a transnational field: A network analysis of the global fact-checking movement. *New Media & Society, 00*, 1–19.

Lemos, A. (2002). *Cibercultura: Tecnologia e Vida Social na Cultura Contemporânea* (1st ed.). Edufba.

Lemos, A. (2020). *Cibercultura: Tecnologia e Vida Social na Cultura Contemporânea* (2nd ed.). Sulina.

Lévy, P. (1997). *Cyberculture*. Odile Jacob.

Lopes, G. (2018). *É verdade que o PT de Haddad distribui mamadeira erótica nas escolas?* [online] E-farsas. Accessed May 7, 2025, from https://www.e-farsas.com/e-verdade-que-o-pt-de-haddad-distribui-mamadeira-erotica-nas-escolas.html

Martel, C., Pennycook, G., & Rand, D. G. (2020). Reliance on emotion promotes belief in fake news. *Cogn Res Princ Implic, 5*, 47.

Modgil, S., Singh, R. K., Gupta, S., et al. (2024). A confirmation bias view on social media induced polarisation during Covid-19. *Information Systems Frontiers, 26*, 417–441.

Moreno-Gil, V., & Salgado-de Dios, F. (2023). El cumplimiento del código de principios de la International Fact-Checking Network en las plataformas de verificación españolas. *Un análisis cualitativo. Revista de Comunicación, 22*(1), 293–307.

Newman, N., Fletcher, R., Robertson, C., et al. (2024). *Reuters Institute Digital News Report 2024*. Reuters Institute for the Study of Journalism.

Nickerson, R. S. (1998). Confirmation bias a ubiquitous phenomenon guises. *Review of General Psychology, 2*(2), 175–220.

Nord, M., Altman, D., Angiolillo, F., et al. (2025). *Democracy Report 2025: 25 years of autocratization – Democracy trumped?* V-Dem Institute.

Pennycook, G., & Rand, D. G. (2018). Lazy, not biased: Susceptibility to partisan fake news is better explained by lack of reasoning than by motivated reasoning. *Cognition, 188*, 39–50.

Pereira Neto, A. (1999). O Estado de São Paulo e a deposição do presidente Goulart (1964): Um estudo sobre as peculiaridades do liberalismo no Brasil. *Revista de História Regional, 4*(2), 107 123.

Portal G1. (2025). *G1 Fato ou Fake - O serviço de checagem de fatos do Grupo Globo*. [online] G1. Accessed May 8, 2025, from https://g1.globo.com/fato-ou-fake/

Preston, S., Anderson, A., Robertson, D. J., et al. (2021). Detecting fake news on Facebook: The role of emotional intelligence. *PLoS ONE, 16*(3), e0246757.

Projeto Comprova. (2018). *'Mamadeiras eróticas' não foram distribuídas em creches pelo PT*. [online] Projeto Comprova. Accessed May 7, 2025, from https://projetocomprova.com.br/post/re_2B5W8XYj0Jwb/

Representação n° 0601530-54.2018.6.00.0000 [2018] (*Ministro Sérgio Banhos*). Accessed May 10, 2025, from https://www.conjur.com.br/dl/de/decisao-tse-fake-news-video-mamadeira.pdf

Rocha, Y. M., De Moura, G. A., Desidério, G. A., et al. (2021). The impact of fake news on social media and its influence on health during the COVID-19 pandemic: A systematic review. *Z Gesundh Wiss - Journal of Public Health*, 1–10.

Statista. (2024). *The Statistics Portal for Market data, Market Research and Market Studies*. [online] Statista.com. Accessed May 10, 2025, from https://www.statista.com/

Stencel, M., Ryan, E., & Luther, J. (2022). *Fact-checkers extend their global reach with 391 outlets, but growth has slowed - Reporters' Lab.* [online] Duke Reporters' Lab. Accessed May 8, 2025, from https://reporterslab.org/2022/06/17/fact-checkers-extend-their-global-reach-with-391-outlets-but-growth-has-slowed/

Stencel, M., Ryan, E., & Luther, J. (2024). *With half the planet going to the polls in 2024, fact-checking sputters - Reporters' Lab.* [online] Reporters' Lab. Accessed May 10, 2025, from https://reporterslab.org/2024/05/30/with-half-the-planet-going-to-the-polls-in-2024-fact-checking-sputters/

Taylor, P. (2024). *Number of smartphone mobile network subscriptions worldwide from 2016 to 2023, with forecasts from 2023 to 2028.* [online] Statista. Accessed May 9, 2025, from https://www.statista.com/statistics/330695/number-of-smartphone-users-worldwide

The Associated Press. (2025a). *AP Fact Check.* [online] AP News. Accessed May 7, 2025, from https://apnews.com/ap-fact-check

The Associated Press. (2025b). *Donate to the Associated Press.* [online] AP News. Accessed May 7, 2025, from https://apnews.com/donate

The Lancet. (2025). Health in the age of disinformation. *The Lancet, 405*(10474), 173.

The Washington Post. (2025). *Fact Checker - The Washington Post.* [online] The Washington Post. Accessed May 9, 2025, from https://www.washingtonpost.com/politics/fact-checker/

Traumann, T. (2020). *Lições do ódio online.* [online] VEJA. Accessed May 10, 2025, from https://veja.abril.com.br/coluna/thomas-traumann/licoes-do-odio-online/

Tribunal Superior Eleitoral. (2018). *Eleições 2018: Justiça Eleitoral conclui totalização dos votos do segundo turno.* [online] Tribunal Superior Eleitoral. Accessed May 9, 2025, from https://www.tse.jus.br/comunicacao/noticias/2018/Outubro/eleicoes-2018-justica-eleitoral-conclui-totalizacao-dos-votos-do-segundo-turno

Udry, J., & Barber, S. J. (2024). The illusory truth effect: A review of how repetition increases belief in misinformation. *Current Opinion in Psychology, 56,* 101736.

University of Gothenburg. (2022). *Dictatorships advancing globally | University of Gothenburg.* [online] University of Gothenburg. Accessed May 10, 2025, from https://www.gu.se/en/news/dictatorships-advancing-globally

Van Dijck, J., Poell, T., & de Waal, M. (2018). *The platform society: Public values in a connective world.* Oxford University Press.

Vinhas, O., & Bastos, M. (2025). When fact-checking is not WEIRD: Negotiating consensus outside western, educated, industrialized, rich, and democratic countries. *The International Journal of Press/Politics, 30*(1), 256–276.

Wardle, C., & Derakhshan, H. (2017). *Information disorder: Toward an interdisciplinary framework for research and policymaking.* Council of Europe.

Zuboff, S. (2019). *The age of surveillance capitalism: The fight for a human future at the new frontier of power.* PublicAffairs.

Index

C
COVID-19, 8, 15–18, 29, 32, 50, 53, 67, 68, 73, 99

D
Digital literacies, 18, 20, 21, 65–77, 96
Disinformation, 1–21, 29, 46, 50, 53, 66–74, 76, 79, 81, 82, 84, 87, 90–93, 97–99

E
Evidence-based medicine (EBM), 42, 43, 47, 53, 54

F
Fake news, 11–18, 28, 69, 70, 84, 85, 94–99

I
Infodemics, 9, 17–20, 29, 50–52, 67, 73, 99
Infodemiology, 17–19, 50

Information and communication technologies (ICTs), 1–5, 7–16, 20, 25, 26, 62–66, 68, 71, 74, 77, 81, 85
Information society, 1–7, 19, 64, 74, 79
Internet, 5, 6, 8, 9, 11–13, 15–17, 20, 25–54, 63, 64, 66, 71, 72, 75, 80, 81, 83, 95

N
Networked society, 62

P
Pandemics, 15–18, 29, 50, 52, 53, 67, 69, 70, 73, 97, 99

S
Social media, 4, 11–13, 16, 17, 19, 28, 52, 70, 84, 92–95, 97, 99

Index

If you have any concerns about our products,
you can contact us on
ProductSafety@springernature.com

In case Publisher is established outside the EU,
the EU authorized representative is:
**Springer Nature Customer Service Center GmbH
Europaplatz 3, 69115 Heidelberg, Germany**

Printed by Libri Plureos GmbH
in Hamburg, Germany